Lymph Taping

The information in this book is intended for medical professionals who have prior knowledge and training of the medical taping method and manual lymphatic treatments. The utmost care has been taken to produce this instruction manual. The author and publisher cannot accept any liability, if, despite this care, the information provided in this manual is incomplete or incorrect. Any suggestions for improvement would be welcomed by the authors. The author and publisher cannot be held liable for the consequences of incorrect, careless or unprofessional application of the treatment described in this manual. Any treatment on a patient with lymph oedema or chronic swelling should be under the direction of a physician. Nobody should use these techniques without the appropriate theoretical and practical knowledge. If there are any concerns, consult the appropriate health care provider. Users of this book are encouraged to confirm the information contained herein with other sources. They are also advised to check the product information sheet included in the package of each material they plan to administer, to be certain that changes have not been made, for example, in contraindications.

Uitgever: Fysionair, www.fysionair.com
Fotografie: Tjerk van der Veen, www.dutch-ceramics.nl
Illustraties: Rogier Trompert, www.medical-art.nl
Omslagontwerp: Zone2 design, www.zone2design.nl
Druk. Looney2 BV, www.looney2.nl
1e druk, oktober 2010
2e druk, juni 2018
ISBN: 978-94-91038-02-0
NUR: 871, 890, 894

LYMPH TAPING

Theory, technique, practice

Josya Sijmonsma

Table of Contents

5. Healthy lymphatic system with temporary overload 85

Foreword

In 2004 the Dutch Medical Taping Concept Manual was published, describing all the techniques of this treatment method. One of the chapters of this book briefly goes into the possibility of influencing lymph drainage with Medical Taping. However, the lymph taping that is described in the Manual, is relatively simple and can only be used with a healthily functioning lymph system.

There was soon found to be a need for a deeper treatment of this subject, which also discussed all the problems of secondary and primary lymph disorders. This book attempts to meet this very need. Advances in understanding have also ensured that the theory regarding the action of lymph taping has had to be thoroughly updated, and this theory can be found in the book.

The cooperation with the Lymph Akademie Deutschland, known for short as L.A.D., has contributed considerably to establishing the improved theory of the action of lymph taping. Thanks are due for this in the first place to Dimitri Reder and Otto Schreiner, both associated with the L.A.D. as specialist teaching staff for MLD/CDPT.

In addition a very large number of people have contributed in various ways to the completion of this book and I would like to thank them at this point. My German colleague Connie Daubert and my Dutch colleague Gerdieke Kastenberg for their inspiring feedback. My Dutch 'mentor from the first hour' Wilma Waters for the basis from which this could arise. Also Marian Franken and Janine Franken for their patient input, Tjerk van der Veen for his aesthetic contribution and Joyce Verhoef from NL Net for her unremitting energy in raising awareness of lymph problems.

The case histories in this book could only take shape because of all the clients and course members who gave their cooperation and consent to use the material for publication. I owe a great deal of thanks to all these people.

The continual enthusiasm of Gert-Jan Olthoff and cooperation with FysioTape has again also been very important to me, not least because of the quality of the CureTape product, with which the treatment results could be achieved.

I would like to thank Klaus Hannken-Illjes because he was the driving force from FoBiZe and L.A.D. for the German-Dutch cooperation.

I would like to express a special word of thanks to Jaap van Barneveld for his patient dedication and for all the times he has encouraged me to complete this project.

I hope that this book will be found to be a valuable addition for all therapists who are faced in their practice with people suffering from any form of lymph problems and above all I hope that in particular these latter people can be better helped by this.

Hof van Twente, 2010

Josya Sijmonsma

1 Introduction

1.1 Medical Taping and Lymph Taping

In around 1970 the base was laid in Asia for a new treatment method. At this time the 'Balance Tape Method' was developed in Korea and a similar 'Kinesio Tape Method' in Japan. These new methods were characterised by the background philosophy and the elastic material worked with.

The basic idea is that muscles are not only necessary for movement, but also play a decisive part for example in blood circulation, lymph drainage and body temperature. If muscles do not function well that may then cause a range of complaints and disorders. For this an elastic tape material was developed, which can effectively support muscle structures in their function, without also limiting movements. In this way the body's own recovery process is stimulated.

The scope is however much wider than just treating muscle structures and up until the present time inventive therapists are discovering new possibilities and indications.

The American Ruth Copee found it was possible to treat specific lymph problems with lymph taping. The possibilities of lymph taping and the special adjunct that this offers in oedema therapy has ensured its rapid acceptance by oedema therapists.

The total treatment method has since the early years of this century been called the *Medical Taping Concept*, the only name for this treatment method that is no longer directly associated with a product name. Lymph taping has become an integral and important part of the total Medical Taping Concept.

1.2 Properties of the tape

The Medical Taping Concept uses CureTape, an elastic, cotton tape with a non-allergenic adhesive layer. The adhesive layer is applied in a special pattern so that the material breathes. As a result the tape is very well tolerated, even when used for long periods. With careful use skin irritation rarely occurs, an aspect which is certainly very important for lymph taping, because even minimal skin irritation can cause an increase in lymphatic pressure.

CureTape can stretch by up to 140%, which is similar to the stretchability of the skin. The thickness and weight of the tape are also similar to the skin. The material is applied to the paper with 10% pretensioning, this pretensioning is used for most tape techniques.

The tape is made of pure cotton, with latex-free elastic fibres woven into it in the longitudinal direction. For this reason the tape can only be stretched in the longitudinal direction, and so is also always used lengthwise.

The adhesive layer absorbs the body heat, and sticks better as the tape warms up. The tape is always lightly massaged into place which warms it up. Once the tape has been massaged into place, it cannot be reused, the tape only sticks once.

CureTape can be worn for several days in a row. Treatment with tape can be carried out for a long time without this causing skin problems. In case of chronic problems, such as primary or secondary lymphoedema, Medical Taping can even be used for years in succession. In case of long term use it is recommended that the tape be replaced once every 5 to 7 days. The tape is water-resistant and withstands showering, swimming or bathing.

1.3 Effects

In most applications of the tape use is made of the stretchability of the tape with respect to the stretchability of the skin. The skin of the area to be treated is stretched by bringing the muscles and joints into a stretched position, the tape is then applied to the skin without stretching.

When the body part returns to its starting position, the elasticity of the tape ensures that the skin is slightly lifted. This creates what are called 'convolutions' which are more or less clearly visible.

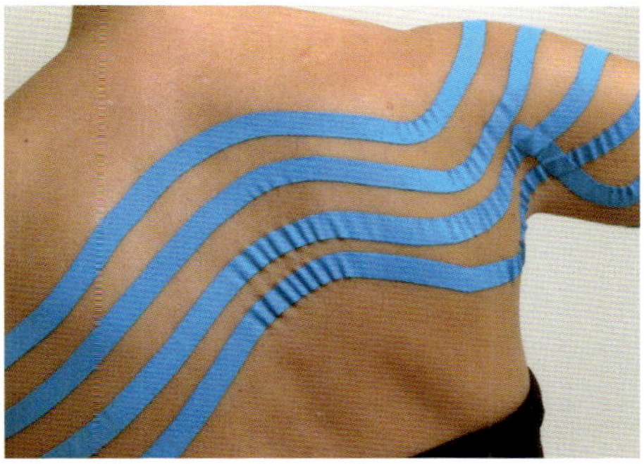

Visible convolutions in a skin area with tape.

More space is then created in the area just under the epidermis, where among other things initial lymph vessels, hair vessels and various afferent and efferent receptors are located.

By using different tape techniques, an effect can be exerted on these different structures or even on the underlying fascia.

To sum up the effects can be broken down as follows:

1. Pain alleviation;
2. Improve muscle function by tone regulation;
3. Support joint function by:
   - stimulating proprioception;
   - influencing position of joints;
   - influencing movement direction;
   - increasing stability.
4. Removing obstructions to lymph drainage;
5. Normalising blood flow;
6. Neuro-reflectory effect.

For a description of these effects and the techniques used, please refer to the general basic book 'Medical Taping Concept – Manual' also published as 'Taping Neuro Muscular – Manual'.
This book 'Lymph Taping' in particular discusses in detail the action and the possible uses in case of lymph problems.

1.4 General points for attention

When using Medical Taping a number of points for attention must be borne in mind:

- The skin should be clean, dry and grease-free.

- It is not a problem to tape over short hairs, as long as the tape adheres to the skin. If there is too much hair, it should be shaved off. Since the tape also has to be removed again, it is in any case recommended that short hairs be removed.

- Certainly in the case of lymph problems, hair should be removed in a skin-friendly way, without using irritants and without the risk of folliculitis. The special small facial trimmers that trim off short hairs are safe to use.

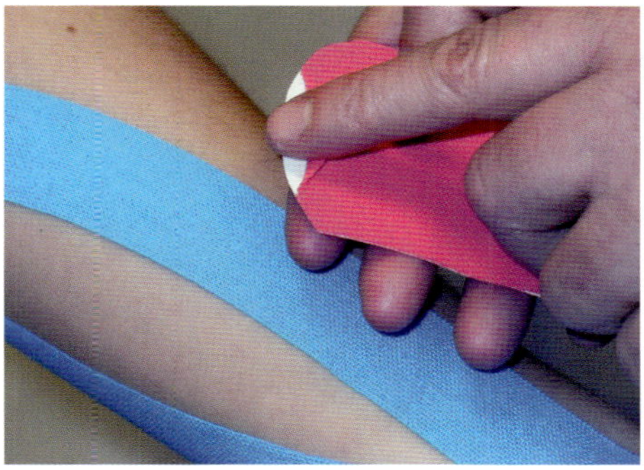

Removing tape from paper.

- To remove the tape from the paper, hold the piece of tape cut off with the cotton side towards you, then with the fingertip pull the top edge at a slight angle.

- Another way of removing the tape from the paper is to tear off a small piece of the paper by the anchor. The tape itself can be stretched and will not tear when you do this.

- The base and the anchor of the tape are always applied without stretching.

- Always cut the corners of the base and anchors of the tape into a round shape, which will help the tape remain in place better and longer.

- Avoid making folds in the tape or in the skin under the tape, skin irritation can easily occur in places with pleats or folds.

- When the tape has been applied, massage it lightly to warm it for optimum adhesion.

- The tape sticks better as the material warms, so take care when applying heat to taped skin areas.

- Sometimes there is short term (10 to 20 minutes) itching under the tape. This is not a problem. In case of itching or irritation that lasts for longer than half an hour, it is recommended that the tape be removed as a precaution.

- The tape should be removed carefully. For preference wet well, stretch the skin tight and roll the tape bit by bit off of the skin. Another possibility is to rub baby oil into the tape and allow this oil to soak in.

- If the tape is not removed with care considerable skin irritation may be caused!

- CureTape can only be used lengthwise. Even the smaller tapes, for example for children, should be cut from the length of the roll.

1.5 Contra indications

The Medical Taping Concept is a recent form of therapy that is still under development. Not a lot is yet known about any contra indications of this method, but on rational grounds and based on facts from experience there are some absolute and relative contra indications to mention.

An absolute contra indication is the inexpert application of the Medical Taping Concept. The therapist should have sufficient factual knowledge of Medical Taping, but also of the pathology to be treated. Lymph Taping in primary or secondary lymphoedema must therefore be reserved for oedema therapists.

The relative contra indications that can be mentioned based on rational considerations are as follows:

- **Thrombosis**
  Medical Taping normalises the circulation, a tape over a thrombus could therefore possibly cause an embolism;

- **Skin defects**
  The tape is not sterile, taping *over* a skin defect is therefore not advised. If the tape is applied *around* the skin defect or wound, the stimulation of the circulation does in fact encourage faster tissue repair;

- **General oedema**
  General oedema because of heart trouble or kidney trouble is a contra indication for manual lymph drainage and therefore also for lymph taping.

- **Carcinomen**
  The presence of carcinomas or metastases in the area to be treated may be a reason to be cautious with manual lymph drainage and/or lymph taping;

- **Fever**
  In case of fever, manual lymph drainage is contra indicated, and so is lymph taping;

- **During the lactation period**
  In case of manual lymph drainage, and also lymph taping, waste products may possibly get into the breast milk;

- **Pregnancy**
  Via the segmental relationship an effect may be exerted on the uterus. Since it is not known at present whether this can affect the pregnancy, caution is called for when applying CureTape over skin areas with a segmental relationship;

- **Irritation or defence mechanism**
  If the tape causes irritation or feels unpleasant, the diagnosis and the technique used should be checked and if necessary adjusted. Especially in the case of lymph taping consideration should be given to whether the lymph strips have been applied from the right drainage area;

- **Skin abnormalities**
  Particularly in the case of a very thin skin the tape should be removed with extra caution!

Diabetes
Diabetes is in principle not a contra indication. In practice however there have been cases where the tape treatment has caused a considerably reduced insulin requirement, especially if tape is applied over parts of the body where the client normally injects the insulin. It is good to be aware of this.

2. Anatomy of the lymphatic system

2.1 Introduction

An exhaustive description of all the anatomical details of the lymphatic system would fill a book on its own. For this reason even as a semblance of completeness, it is scarcely possible in this book to suggest that it covers the anatomy of the lymphatic system.

It is not therefore intended to give an exhaustive anatomical description here. An attempt has however been made to summarise the anatomical aspects where these are relevant to give an overall idea of the anatomy of the lymphatic system. The choices that are necessary for this summary have mainly been made with the objective of explaining why lymph taping deserves a clear place within the therapeutic process.

For a fuller description of the anatomy of the lymphatic system please refer to the textbooks on lymphology or lymph drainage.

2.1.1 The circulation system

The total circulation in the body consists of the blood circulation, divided into the arterial system and the venous system, with in addition the lymphatic system.

The lymphatic system is a draining system which runs in parallel to the venous part of the blood circulation.
The circulation can be divided into a 'high pressure system' and a 'low pressure system'.

The arterial system is the high pressure system, the venous system together with the lymphatic system forms the low pressure system.

Via the lymph vessels and the lymph nodes the lymphatic system ultimately passes into the venous system at the point where the venous pressure is the lowest, close to the heart.

There are many similarities between the blood circulation system and the draining lymphatic system, for example a similar vascular structure and a similar distribution in the body, but there are also clear differences. The lymphatic system is not a closed system, but only drains lymph. Another difference is that the lymphatic system has no central pump.

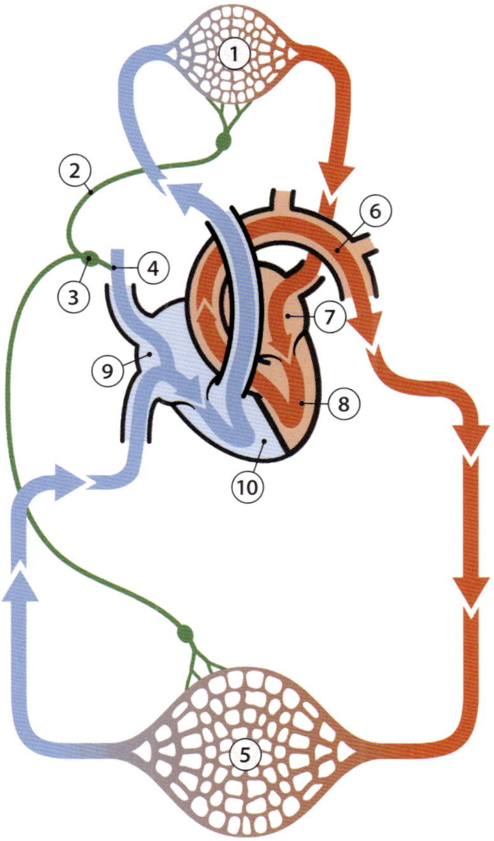

1. Microcirculation lung
2. Lymph vessel
3. Lymph node
4. Venous angle
5. Microcirculation
6. Aorta
7. Left atrium
8. Left ventricle
9. Right atrium
10. Right ventricle

2.1.2 Function of the lymphatic system

Around 80 to 90 % of the fluid pushed from the blood circulation into the interstitium is then reabsorbed by the venous system. The remaining 10 to 20 % of the fluid is absorbed and drained by the lymphatic system. As soon as the interstitial fluid is absorbed by the lymph vessels, this fluid is called lymph.
Apart from water small molecular substances and proteins also leave the bloodstream. The small molecular substances are reabsorbed by the venous system, but the proteins cannot be reabsorbed by the veins and are drained via the lymphatic system.
In addition the lymphatic system removes harmful substances that may be present in the body. In short, the lymphatic system removes all the substances that cannot or may not pass into the bloodstream. These are called the 'lymph-dependent substances'.
The total volume of lymph-dependent substances and water is the lymphatic load.
The lymphatic load is filtered and purified in the intermediate lymph nodes, after which the purified lymph is absorbed back into the bloodstream.

2.1.3 Lymphatic organs

These form part of the immune system and have a function in detecting, fighting and rendering harmless pathogens, exogenous cells and proteins and malignant degenerate cells.
The lymphatic organs are subdivided into the primary lymphatic organs and the secondary lymphatic organs. The primary lymphatic organs consist of the red bone marrow and the thymus.
In the red bone marrow the lymphocytes are made. The lymphocytes are subdivided into the T-lymphocytes which leave the bone marrow early on to mature further in the thymus, and the B-lymphocytes which develop further in the bone marrow.
The main secondary lymphatic organs are the lymph nodes and the spleen, but also include the tonsils for example.

2.1.4 Lymph nodes

The lymph nodes, or nodi lymphatici, are often (incorrectly) called the 'lymph glands'. These filter stations are located in a network along the lymph vessels, usually embedded in fatty tissue. The form, number and size of these lymph nodes vary considerably.

The total number of lymph nodes is already present at birth and usually varies between 600 to 700. The size depends on the constitution, age, functional load and total number of lymph nodes present. In adults the lymph nodes are between the 0.2 cm and 3 cm in size. Very enlarged lymph nodes usually indicate pathological changes.

Although lymph nodes may increase or even decrease in size during the lifetime, the total number of lymph nodes does not change under normal conditions. If lymph nodes are lost for example due to surgical procedures, they do not regenerate.

Lymph flows into the lymph nodes via afferent vessels and leaves the lymph nodes via the efferent vessels. The entry of the often branched afferent vessels is spread over the surface of the lymph nodes. The efferent vessels leave the lymph node at the hilum.

The efferent vessels are less numerous compared with the afferent vessels, have a larger diameter and contain more valves.

The afferent vessels may be lymph collectors from the periphery, or internodal lymph vessels – that is an efferent vessel from another lymph node. In this way different lymph nodes are connected to one another and form a network.

To ensure sufficient purification of the lymph, the lymph usually flows through several lymph nodes before flowing back into the venous circulation.

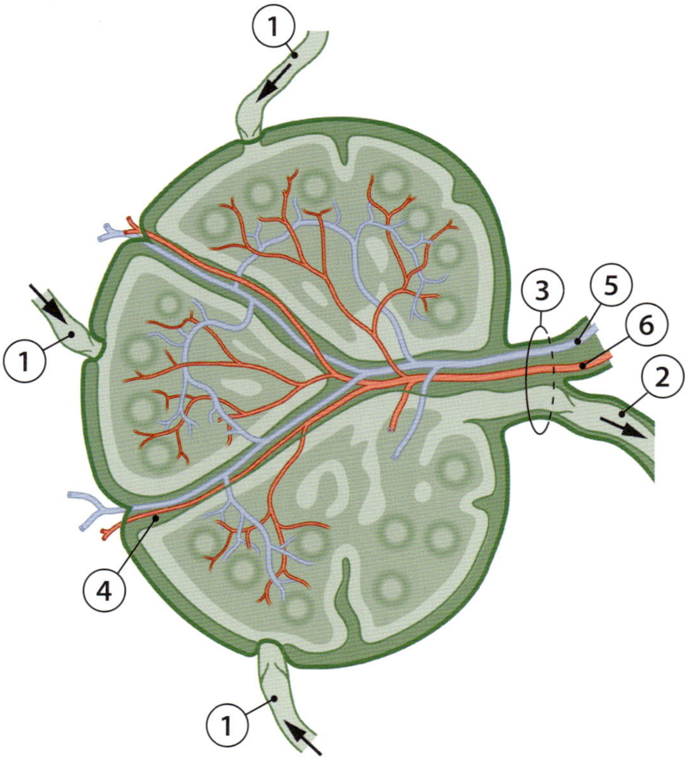

1. Afferent lymph vessels
2. Efferent lymph vessels
3. Hilum
4. Trabeculae
5. Vein
6. Artery

The capsule of a lymph node is composed of collagen tissue with some elastic fibres and smooth muscle tissue between them.
From the hilum the lymph node is divided into open compartments by trabeculae. In these trabeculae the larger blood vessels of the lymph node also flow. Between the trabeculae large numbers of lymphocytes and macrophages are also present.

In the lymph nodes blood and lymph flow in parallel, as a result of which exchange of cellular and non-cellular elements can take place. Also a large proportion of the water present in the lymph flow is absorbed by the blood vessels.
In the lymph nodes antibodies are formed, which can be absorbed directly by the blood.

The rate at which the lymph circulates through the lymph node is considerably lower than the rate in the lymph vessels, as a result of which the macrophages present have the optimum opportunity to detect harmful substances and render them harmless.

The lymph nodes therefore have multiple functions:

- filtering the lymph brought in;
- the lymphocytes render antigens in the lymph harmless;
- producing antibodies;
- condensing lymph fluid.

2.2 Prelymphatic channels and lymph vessels

The total lymphatic system consists of a prelymphatic part and a lymphatic part. A characteristic of the lymphatic part is that it is bounded by endothelium.

The prelymphatic part consists of interstitial channels in the intercellular space, which are not bounded by endothelium. These prelymphatic channels pass through cell bulges and elastic connective tissue (that have a sort of conducting function) to the initial lymph vessels. An important aspect here is that the prelymphatic channels of the skin and the subcutis *do not* respect the lymphatic watershed (see also § 2.3.2).

The lymphatic part of the lymphatic system is an efferent one-way system of converging vessels, which is similar in structure to the venous system. The lymphatic system begins in the periphery with the initial lymph vessels or the lymph capillaries. Specific for the lymphatic system are the intermediate lymph nodes.

Based on their wall structure, lymph vessels are sub-divided into:

- lymph capillaries or initial lymph vessels;
- precollectors;
- collectors;
- lymph stems.

The lymph stems ultimately lead into the venous system via the vena subclavia and the vena jugularis interna, or the right and left venous angle.

The total lymphatic system can be subdivided into three related parts:

1. The surface or subcutaneous system which provides the drainage of skin and subcutis;
2. The deep or subfascial system which provides the drainage of muscles, joints and nerves;
3. The organ system which provides the drainage of the different organs.

The surface and the deep system are connected to one another via small vessels. Most of these small connecting vessels carry lymph from the deep system to the surface system.

2.2.1 Initial lymph vessels

The lymphatic system begins with a fine network of initial lymph vessels that are embedded in the interstitial connective tissue. Depending on the degree of filling the diameter of an initial lymph vessel may increase to 1 mm. The initial lymph vessels have no valve system.

The initial lymph vessels contain bulges, where at certain points the endothelium cells partly overlap one another. These overlapping edges may move apart from one another. In this way a sort of 'inlet valve' is formed, through which fluid from the interstitium can enter the lymphatic system.

Level with these 'inlet valves' anchor filaments are attached that are connected with the collagen and elastic fibres of the interstitium. These elastic fibres also act as a conductor for tissue fluid and hence form a pre-lymphatic pathway.

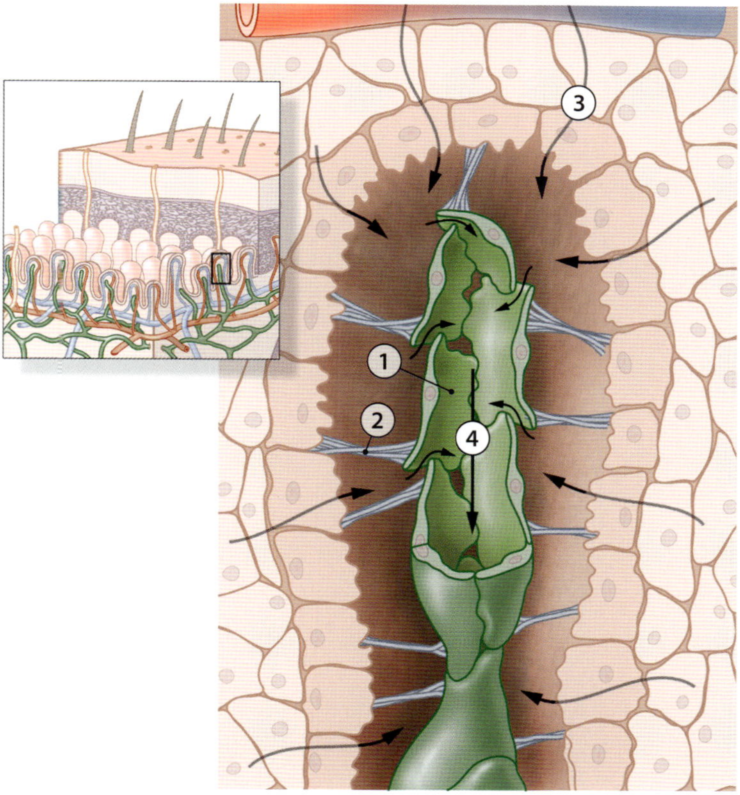

1. *Endothelium cells*
2. *Anchor filaments*
3. *Direction prelymphatic fluid*
4. *Direction lymph flow*

2.2.2 Precollectors

From the initial lymph vessels the lymph flows to the slightly wider precollectors that have a diameter of around 1.5 mm. The precollectors contain both segments with characteristics of the initial vessels, and segments with characteristics of the collectors into which they flow.

Some segments have the 'inlet valves' as in the initial lymph vessels. The precollectors therefore have a share in the absorption of fluid.

Other segments already contain some smooth muscle tissue in the wall like that found in the collectors. The precollectors also have valves here and there to prevent backflow, but less numerous than in the collectors. These characteristics support the transport function of the precollectors.

2.2.3 Collectors

The collectors collect lymph from the precollectors to then transport lymph to the lymph nodes and lymph stems. The diameter of the collectors varies between 0.1 and 0.6 mm.

The structure of the vessel walls of the collectors is similar to the structure of the vessel walls of the veins; the vessel walls of a collector also contain smooth muscle tissue.
Valves are present in the collectors that prevent the backflow of lymph fluid. The valves lie at irregular distances from one another, the distance between the valves may vary from 6 to 20 mm.

The part of the collector which lies between a distal pair and a proximal pair of valves is called a lymphangion. A lymphangion forms a functional unit which can contract due to the presence of smooth muscle tissue in the wall. The succession of lymphangions in this way produces a peristaltic movement which pumps the lymph further.

The surface collectors roughly follow the path of the larger skin veins and therefore run in relatively straight lines. A collector has a number of spread out collaterals, which form a bridge for part of the route. The collaterals can hence relieve or replace part of the collector.
Collectors are connected to one another by anastomoses through which the lymph can flow to a collector in another area. These anastomoses have valves at the beginning, so that the lymph can only flow to proximal.

2.2.4 Trunci lymphatici of lymfestammen

The lymph ultimately flows from the lymph nodes and the collectors via the lymph stems (trunci lymphatici) to the right and the left venous angle. The drainage from the top right quadrant of the body passes via the right venous angle, the other three body quadrants drain to the left venous angle.

The left and right lumbar stem (truncus lumbalis sinister and truncus lumbalis dexter) provide the lymph drainage from the lower half of the body.
The truncus gastrointestinales drains lymph from stomach, intestines, liver and pancreas. These three stems lead into the cisterna chyli, a sort of reservoir in which the clear lymph from the legs and the cloudier lymph from the truncus gastrointestinales flow together.

From the cisterna chyli the biggest lymph stem of the body, the ductus thoracicus, carries the lymph further to proximal. The ductus thoracicus passes through the diaphragm level with the hiatus aortica to ultimately flow into the left venous angle.
The truncus subclavius sinister and the truncus jugularis sinister also pass into the left venous angle.

The left venous angle consists of the left v. jugularis interna and the left v. subclavia. The valves present at this connection point ensure that no venous blood can flow back into the lymphatic system.

In the right venous angle three lymph stems merge: the truncus jugularis dexter, the truncus subclavius dexter and the truncus bronchomediastinalis.

Drainage area of the lymph stems:

Truncus lumbalis	lymph drainage of the legs, abdomen and skin below the navel.
Truncus gastrointestinales	lymph drainage of stomach, intestines, liver and pancreas.
Ductus thoracicus	starts in the cisterna chyli, leading into the left venous angle.
Truncus subclavius	lymph drainage of arm, shoulder and skin above the navel.
Truncus jugularis	lymph drainage from the head and neck area.
Truncus bronchomediastinalis	lymph drainage chest (except for the skin), and partly from heart and lungs.

It should also be noted that there are many anatomical variations in the layout of lymph stems.

2.3 The subcutaneous lymph drainage system

The surface or subcutaneous lymphatic system provides the drainage of skin and subcutis, while the deep or subfascial system provides the drainage of muscles, joints and nerves.
These systems are connected to one another via connecting vessels or anastomoses. Most of these anastomoses carry the lymph from the deep system to the surface system.

The surface system is divided into skin territories. A skin territory is composed of different skin zones, a skin zone comprises a number of skin areas.

2.3.1 Areas, zones and territories

The skin region that is drained by initial lymph vessels that connect to a single precollector is called a skin area. Because skin areas partly overlap one another, the lymph from the region of an area may in fact drain in different directions.

The different skin areas of which the precollectors flow into one collector, together form a skin zone. Skin zones are connected to one another via the overlapping skin areas of which they are composed and by numerous anastomoses with neighbouring collectors. Through these connections lymph can be drained in several flow directions.

All the skin zones together of which the collectors lead into one collector bundle, form a skin territory. Because territories have far fewer anastomoses with one another, the edges of the territories form a sort of 'boundary', called the watershed.

2.3.2 Watersheds

The skin of the trunk can be subdivided into eight territories. The vertical watershed is formed by the median line, while the horizontal watershed runs between the navel and the processus spinosus of the second lumbar vertebra. A vertical line from the armpit forms the watershed between the ventral and dorsal territories.

The crista iliaca and the ligament inguinale form a watershed between the lower extremity and the trunk. In the cranium there is a watershed between the trunk and the cervical section that runs ventrally over the claviculae and dorsally over the spinae scapulae.
Skin territories can also be separated from one another by watersheds in the upper and lower extremities.

Although the skin territories have few anastomoses with one another, the watersheds are bridged by the surface network of overlapping skin areas and connected skin zones. As a result there is always a possibility that the lymph from a particular territory is drained via an adjacent territory.

1. *Watersheds*
2. *Vena cava superior*
3. *Ductus thoracicus*
4. *Cisterna chyli*
5. *Truncus jugularis*
6. *Truncus subclavius*
7. *Axillary lymph nodes*
8. *Truncus bronchomediastinalis*
9. *Truncus gastrointestinales*
10. *Truncus lumbalis*
11. *Inguinal lymph nodes*

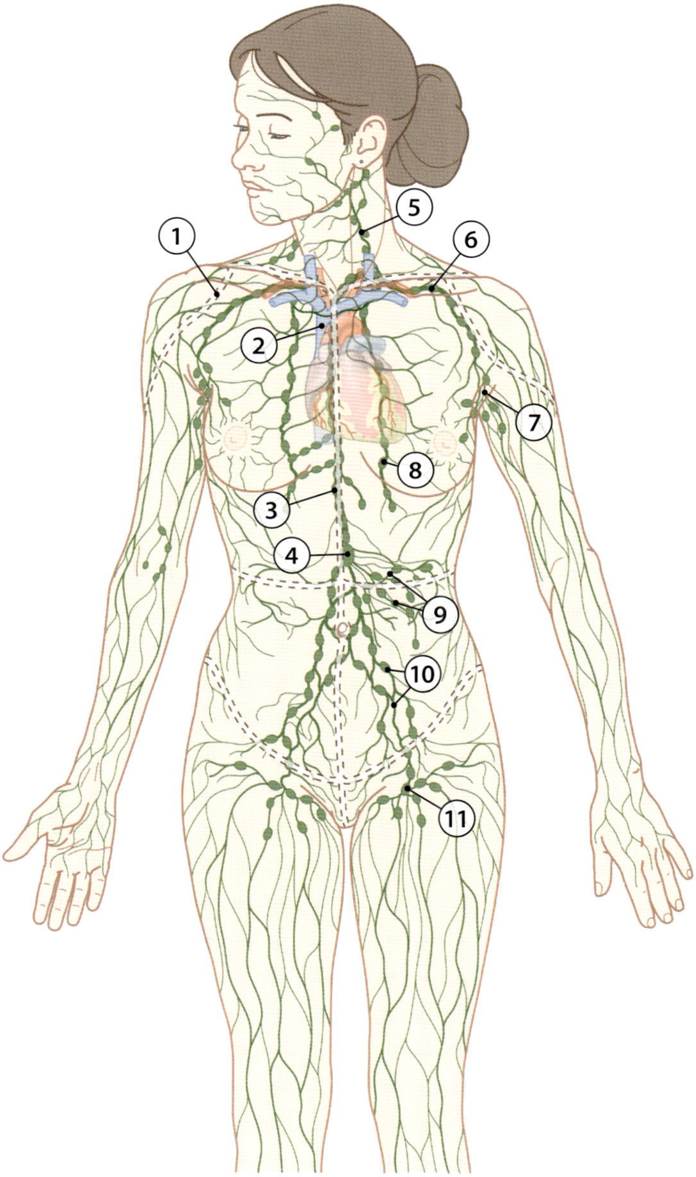
1
2
3
4
5
6
7
8
9
10
11

2.3.3 Anastomoses and alternative routes

Connecting vessels or anastomoses within the lymphatic system guarantee the drainage of lymph at various levels. First of all there are the numerous anastomoses between the subcutaneous (surface) and the subfascial (deep) lymphatic system. The skin zones of which the skin territories are composed also have many anastomoses with one another. Skin areas of initial lymph vessels overlap with one another and bridge the watershed.

In the case of lymph congestion or lymphostasis, various alternative routes are possible for lymph drainage:

- Due to lymph congestion the lymph vessels are overfilled, as a result of which the pressure within the collectors and precollectors increases. If the pressure in the direction of flow is higher than in the afferent lymph vessels, the lymph will flow back to the initial lymph vessels (=dermal backflow). The lymph can then be drained via another pathway where the pressure is lower. In this way the watershed can be bypassed.

- Abnormal widening of lymph collectors can cause a valve insufficiency. This can give a retrograde lymph flow from the overfilled area to a territory where the lymphatic pressure is lower. These are called the interterritorial anastomoses. The most important are the interaxillary anastomoses, the interinguinal anastomoses and the axillo-inguinal anastomoses.

3. Physiology and pathophysiology

3.1 Introduction

For this chapter the same choice has been made as for the previous chapter. The physiology of blood circulation and lymph transport is a very extensive and complex subject. An attempt is therefore made to summarise this into the most relevant details within the subject of this book: lymph taping.
For a more detailed description of this subject please refer to the textbooks on lymphology, lymph drainage or physiology.

3.2 Circulation and blood pressure

One of the functions of the lymphatic system is to drain fluid from the tissue. This is closely related with the blood circulation in the body. The lymphatic system together with the venous system forms part of the low pressure system, while the arterial system forms the high pressure system.

The blood volume that flows through a blood vessel is determined by the difference in pressure at the start and end of the segment, together with the flow resistance. The flow resistance comes about due to a combination of different factors: the viscosity of the fluid, the length of the vessel and the diameter of the vessel. The narrower the blood vessel, the higher the flow resistance, so the smaller the blood volume flowing through the vessel.

From the heart the blood is pumped into the aorta at an average pressure of around 100 mmHg. The flow resistance is low there, as a result of which the blood pressure in the arteries may still be 85 mmHg. The peripheral resistance of the arterial system is mainly determined by the precapillary arterioles, which have a diameter of only 4-25 micrometres. With the same blood volume that therefore means a considerable increase in the flow resistance when the blood goes to the arterioles, and the blood pressure here drops to around 30 mmHg.
The diameter of the capillaries is 5 to 9 micrometres, the viscosity of the blood in these small vessels is a more important factor for determining the

flow resistance. The viscosity is not only determined by the erythrocytes present, but also by the leucocytes, even if these are inactive. If the leucocytes and hence the endothelial cells of the blood capillaries are activated, then the peripheral resistance increases even more.
At the venous end of a blood capillary the pressure has as a result fallen to around 10 mmHg, in the direction of the vena cava the pressure falls even further to ultimately 0 mmHg.

3.2.1 Vasomotion

The flow resistance therefore has a considerable effect on the blood pressure in the precapillary arterioles. In addition the precapillary arterioles also by their own pulsation, independent of the heart, affect the blood pressure in the capillaries. This pulsation, with a frequency of around 10 per minute, is called 'vasomotion'.
Vasomotion is primarily regulated by the oxygen concentration in the tissue. If the oxygen concentration in the tissue decreases, then the frequency of vasomotion falls, as a result of which oxygen goes to the tissue.
The precapillary arterioles have ample smooth musculature in the wall, the postcapillary venules have only sparse smooth musculature in the vessel wall. The nerve supply to the smooth musculature is by the sympaticus, this ensures a resting tone of the smooth musculature which determines the diameter of the vessel.
Increase in the sympaticus activity causes vaso-constriction, as a result of which the capillary blood flow decreases and the pressure in the vessel falls. During vaso-dilation the blood capillary pressure rises and the blood flow of the capillaries increases. This is an active hyperaemia.
Passive hyperaemia is caused by insufficient venous drainage, for example as a result of cardiac insufficiency or pregnancy. Due to venous stasis a pressure increase occurs within the vessel, as a result of which the vessel widens.
Variations in capillary blood pressure may seriously affect lymphoedema present.

3.2.2 Transport

The exchange of substances occurs mainly in the very smallest vessels, the capillaries. Blood capillaries have a permeable wall; supply and drainage of substances occurs here primarily by diffusion.

Diffusion: *transport of substances dissolved in water or gas from a region with a high concentration of these substances to a region with a lower concentration, until equilibrium is reached. This is passive transport that takes no energy.*

Osmosis: *is in fact diffusion of the solvent through a semi-permeable wall. Water molecules move from a place with a greater number of water molecules to a place with a lower number of water molecules. The semi-permeable wall does let water molecules through, but other substances cannot pass through this wall. This process also continues until equilibrium is reached.*

Osmotic transport takes place under the effect of osmotic pressure. The osmotic pressure is determined by the concentration of the molecules present. The more concentrated the solution, the higher the osmotic pressure.
The hydrostatic pressure (or fluid pressure) rises in the area of the concentrated solution, because the water molecules move towards it. Equilibrium occurs when the hydrostatic pressure difference compensates for the difference in osmotic value.

Plasma proteins are macromolecules which are too big to pass through the semi-permeable membrane. These plasma proteins are called colloids. The process of osmosis creates colloid-osmotic pressure which is proportionate to the protein concentration. If the concentration of proteins falls, then the colloid-osmotic pressure falls.

3.3 Physiology of the lymphatic system

A number of important functions of the lymphatic system are: drainage of interstitial fluid, drainage of proteins and drainage of harmful substances. Under normal conditions the maximum transport capacity of the lymphatic system is 10 to 20 times higher than the volume that is actually transported.
Because the lymphatic system under normal, physiological conditions only works at 5 to 10 % of the maximum capacity, there is an enormous functional reserve. Because of this physiological protection it is possible for the lymphatic system to respond adequately to a volume increase of the lymphatic load, without oedema occurring.
This safety mechanism has a passive and an active component.

Passive protection
An increase in the volume of water leaving the blood capillaries causes an increase in the volume of water in the interstitium. The interstitial pressure rises, which ensures that the filtration of water from the capillaries falls.

The extra water in the interstitium lowers the protein concentration in the interstitium, which reduces the colloid osmotic pressure. As a result more fluid is absorbed by the capillaries.

Active protection
The lymphatic system responds to an increase in the volume of water in the interstitium by an increased uptake. The rising pressure in the interstitium causes a tractive force on the anchor filaments of the initial lymph vessels, which causes the 'inlet valves' to open. Because the pressure in the lumen of the lymph capillary is lower than the pressure in the interstitium, the lymphatic load moves from the interstitium to the lumen of the lymph vessel.
This flow continues until the lumen is filled to the maximum. In this phase the pressure in the lumen is even higher than the interstitial pressure.
Due to the pressure difference the 'inlet valves' close. Because the flow resistance in the direction of the precollectors, that have a slightly larger diameter, is lower, the lymph will normally flow in this direction.

At the same time as the increased absorption, the frequency of contraction of smooth muscle tissue in the collectors and the lymph stems rises due to the increase in the intralymphatic pressure. In this way (a part of) the functional reserve of the lymphatic system can be activated.
Increase of the protein concentration in the tissue activates this protection too. More protein causes an increase in the colloid osmotic pressure, which causes more water to leave the capillaries. In total this gives the same effect.

As long as the transport capacity of the lymphatic system exceeds the volume of the lymphatic load, the lymphatic system is functional and no oedema occurs.

3.3.1 Insufficiency of the lymphatic system

As soon as the volume of the lymphatic load becomes greater than the transport capacity of the lymphatic system, an accumulation of fluid or oedema occurs. Oedema in this meaning of the word is a symptom which may be based on various causes.
Insufficiency of the lymphatic system is divided into three groups:

Dynamic insufficiency
In this form there is an anatomically and functionally intact lymphatic system, but the volume of the lymphatic load is greater than the transport capacity. Therefore the functional reserve of the lymphatic system is also already used up. This is also called a 'high output failure'. A low protein oedema occurs in the interstitium.
Because the lymphatic system here is intact and its maximum capacity is already used up, it is not sensible to try to prevent this oedema using measures that are intended to increase the transport. The therapeutic intervention must be aimed at reducing the lymphatic load.

In other words, this form of oedema is *not an indication* for manual lymph drainage or lymph taping.

Dynamic insufficiency can for example arise in case of:
- Cardiac insufficiency;
- Renal insufficiency;
- Chronic venous insufficiency;
- Thrombophlebitis;
- Disturbed protein balance in the tissue.

Mechanical insufficiency
This involves a normal lymphatic load, but due to organic or functional causes the transport capacity of the lymphatic system is reduced as a result of which the whole volume of the lymphatic load cannot be drained. This is also called a 'low output failure'. A protein rich oedema occurs in the interstitium. This oedema is a lymphoedema.

Because the pressure in the lymphatic system rises here, the vessel walls of the lymphangions can become fibrous. In addition in the long term tissue damage will occur due to the accumulation of water, proteins and waste products in the interstitium.

In case of mechanical insufficiency the therapeutic intervention can be aimed at improving lymph transport. In other words, manual lymph drainage and lymph taping are indicated here.

Possible causes for the occurrence of mechanical insufficiency:

- Primary lymphoedema (a congenital disorder of the lymphatic system, see also § 3.4.1);
- Surgical intervention;
- Radiotherapy;
- Traumata;
- Inflammations;
- Toxic paralysis of the lymph vessels;
- Valve insufficiency due to dilation of the lymph vessels.

Combined dynamic and mechanical insufficiency

Here the transport capacity of the lymphatic system is reduced, while at the same time the volume of the lymphatic load is increased. This situation can lead to severe tissue damage (ulcera).

It may be clear that both in case of mechanical insufficiency and in case of dynamic insufficiency a combined insufficiency may occur.

In this 'Lymph Taping' book the treatment of lymphoedema as a result of mechanical insufficiency is further developed.

3.4 Lymphoedema

Lymphoedema is a commonly occurring, serious and chronic condition that can have far-reaching consequences. These consequences have already frequently been played down in medical circles. This is logical in view of the fact that lymphoedema is still poorly identified and recognised by professional practitioners.

Untreated lymphoedema is progressive, so in the long term serious tissue damage can occur. Lymphoedema may be accompanied by various complications, such as fibrosis, lymphangitis, lymphorrhoea and cellulitis. Psychosocially the presence of lymphoedema is very damaging.

As described in the previous paragraph, lymphoedema arises in case of mechanical insufficiency of the lymphatic system. The transport capacity of the lymphatic system is reduced, while the lymphatic load is physiological. This lymphoedema is divided into two categories, namely secondary or acquired lymphoedema, and primary or congenital lymphoedema.

Secondary lymphoedema is the most generally known, most therapists know this as a complication after a mastectomy where axillary node dissection has also been carried out. It is much less generally known that such secondary oedema can also arise after other forms of cancer in which lymph nodes have been removed, though it is a similar pathology.

The situation for primary lymphoedema is even more distressing. Certainly in the Netherlands, this clinical picture is very poorly identified and recognised. Many therapists do not even know primary lymphoedema as a diagnosis.

3.4.1 Primary lymphoedema

Primary lymphoedema is a congenital abnormality, where the lymphatic system does not have a sufficiently functional lay-out. There are various forms of primary lymphoedema, including a number of hereditary forms. Although it is a congenital abnormality, lymphoedema does not have to be already present immediately after birth. The lymphatic system by its very nature after all has a big functional reserve, and as long as this reserve is sufficient to transport the quantity of lymph supplied, there will be no symptoms of lymphoedema.
However as soon as the functional reserve is exhausted, lymphoedema will manifest itself. This can in principle be at any age. Sometimes this happens without a clear trigger factor, it may also be that a minimal trauma is a trigger factor.
The fact that primary lymphoedema can develop spontaneously at any age is explained by the long term overload of the system. There are many factors that may affect the volume of the lymphatic load, which could also explain why lymphoedema may (apparently) suddenly become evident.

Factors affecting the lymphatic load

1. Temperature
   At higher temperatures vasodilation occurs, so more water passes from the blood vessels to the interstitium;
2. Infections
   In the case of infections an increased lymphocyte activity occurs;
3. Too much activity
   If proportionately too much muscular action is carried out, vasodilation occurs;
4. Passivity
   The muscle pump mechanism no longer helps with the drainage;
5. Tissue damage or sterile inflammations
   The histamine released causes vasodilation;
6. Stress
   Reduces the lymph motor function.

Except for the points mentioned, there are probably a lot more factors that affect the volume of the lymphatic load. For example foods, additives, air humidity, air pressure, air load etc.

Although primary lymphoedema may occur anywhere in the body, the lower extremities are usually the biggest problem. This does not have to be symmetrical, the presentation depends on the abnormality in the lymphatic system.

There may be hypoplasia, where the number of lymph vessels involved is reduced, often here the diameter of the lymph vessels is also less than normal.
In case of hyperplasia the diameter of the collectors is too big, so that the valve system is insufficient, which may give rise to a lymph reflux. In case of aplasia part of the lymphatic system is completely absent. Complete aplasia is not compatible with life.

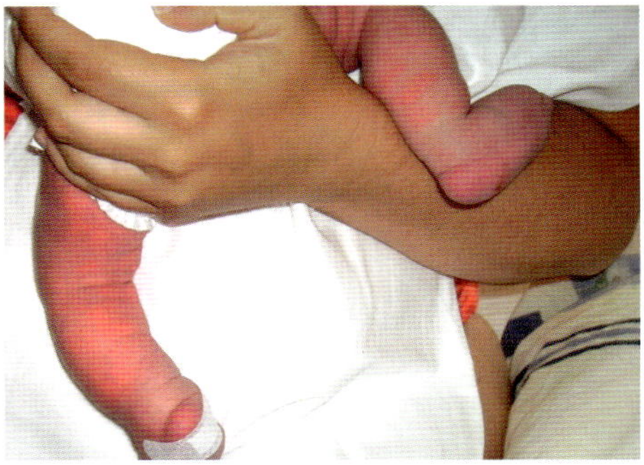

Baby with primary lymphoedema due to Turner syndrome, see §7.3.

Primary lymphoedema is often classified by the age at which the symptoms appear:

Congenital: lymphoedema develops within two years after birth;
Lymphoedema praecox: develops during puberty and adolescence;
Lymphoedema tarda: develops after the age of 35.

In all cases more women than men are involved.

Primary lymphoedema praecox, where the lymphoedema becomes manifest in puberty or as an adolescent, is the most common. Now lymphoedema, the causes and trigger factors have been clarified, it will also be clear why in the previous paragraph primary lymphoedema is called a 'distressing situation'.

This is caused by compounding a number of views and ideas:
1. Primary lymphoedema as stated is very poorly identified and recognised.
2. At the present time the ideal image is to be slim.
3. The modern view within healthcare is that virtually all clinical pictures improve as a result of more exercise.
4. Overweight is seen as the biggest threat to health and according to the modern view should mainly be countered by more exercise.

What happens when a girl at puberty begins to get symptoms due to developing lymphoedema (or lipoedema, see § 3.5.1) as a result of a congenital abnormality in the lymphatic system hardly needs describing. This adolescent starts to suffer from heavy, tired legs. If she goes to her doctor or physiotherapist with these symptoms, the therapist's solution will be obvious. More exercise. If she then in fact actually does play a lot of sport, the lymphatic load can increase further due to vasodilation.
Her legs therefore become thicker, in this case. Because she will want to conform with peer pressure, the response to a disproportionate increase in size is clear. But the conclusion is already drawn too easily that she must lose weight. She must therefore take more exercise and in particular eat less. If she unfortunately also follows a diet here in which the protein intake is restricted, then her situation will get even worse due to the upset protein balance.
If she goes back to a doctor or physiotherapist, all too often they still do not identify and therefore do not recognise the primary lymphoedema. It is more likely that the therapist simply does not believe that she is training so hard and is on such a severe diet. The advice will be to take more exercise and follow a diet. Whereupon the girl has landed in a morbid vicious circle.
It should however be noted that *not* exercising, passivity, also does not help the situation. The muscle pump mechanism supports lymph drainage.

The condition can certainly not be called rare. Because this is not an officially registered disease, no precise figures are known. The estimates of the researchers therefore vary widely, furthermore the studies are poorly comparable due to the different populations and the differences in inclusion and exclusion criteria. A frequently quoted publication is the "Bonn Vein Study", which looked at the occurrence of a positive Stemmer's sign (see § 3.4.4) that is seen as virtually proving the presence of lymphoedema. In this study a positive Stemmer's sign was found in 17.2% of the women and 14.6% of the men (3.2% under 20 years). Stemmer's sign is of course also positive for a secondary lymphoedema.

The identification of lymphoedema and primary lymphoedema is relatively simple. See for this § 3.4.4.

3.4.2 Secondary lymphoedema

Secondary lymphoedema is an acquired lymphoedema, where it is clear what has caused the damage to the lymphatic system. As already stated before, the lymphoedema that can occur after a mastectomy in which the lymph nodes in the armpit are also removed, is the best known. There are however more causes for the occurrence of secondary lymphoedema.

In all other procedures in which lymph nodes are removed, lymphoedema can also occur in the part of the body from which the lymph drainage via these lymph nodes would normally run.

The removal of (some of) the lymph nodes means a reduction in the transport capacity of the lymphatic system. Lymphoedema occurs if the volume of the lymphatic load is greater than the remaining transport capacity. Lymphoedema will not occur as long as the transport capacity is sufficient. The removal of lymph nodes does not therefore unavoidably have to cause lymphoedema in view of the big functional reserve that is normally present.

Radiotherapy causes skin damage, in which tissue may become fibrotic. This has a negative effect on the transport capacity of the lymphatic system.

Infections in which lymph nodes (lymphadenitis) or lymph collectors (lymphangitis) are involved, can lead to fibrosis of the walls of the lymph vessel, which reduces the transport capacity. A complication in Rheumatoid Arthritis may be that the joint infection spreads to the lymphatic system, which can give rise to lymphoedema.

Injuries in which a lot of skin is damaged, such as for example in case of burns, can have an impact on the transport capacity of the lymphatic system, which can give rise to lymphoedema. The scar tissue can make it difficult for the lymph vessels to regenerate, so the situation gets even worse.

Note that posttraumatic secondary lymphoedema is not the same as a posttraumatic oedema. The first is the result of damage to the lymphatic system, the second is a local problem which usually disappears again within a relatively short time.

Filariasis, a parasitic infection, is a major cause of secondary lymphoedema worldwide. The parasite is transferred from person to person by mosquitoes, and causes an infection in the lymphatic system. Filariasis occurs in large parts of Africa and Asia, and also in part of South America.

In all the above-mentioned causes of secondary lymphoedema, it may of course be that an underlying, but not yet manifest, primary lymphoedema complicates the situation or is even the reason for the lymphoedema occurring.

Secondary oedema also does not have to develop immediately. There may be a latency time of many years in which the functional reserve of the lymphatic system is still sufficient to prevent lymphoedema occurring. The explanation for this latency time is the same as described in the previous paragraph: the long term overload and the many, complex interrelated, factors that may affect the volume of the lymphatic load.

3.4.3 Grades of lymphoedema

Lymphoedema as a result of mechanical insufficiency virtually always develops progressively if it is not adequately treated. The lymphatic system is damaged, causing the transport capacity to become insufficient. The prelymphatic fluid which can no longer be adequately drained gradually accumulates in the interstitium.
A distinction is made between different stages:

<u>Latent stage</u>
In this stage the transport capacity of the lymphatic system is of course reduced, but the functional reserve is still sufficient to be able to drain the total lymphatic load. This causes a reduction in the functional reserve, where it depends on the circumstances and the size of the residual capacity whether (and if so, when) lymphoedema will develop.

<u>First stage</u>
In this stage the tissue is still soft, no irreparable tissue damage has occurred. This is also called the reversible stage. Pitting oedema occurs, in other words, the pressure of a thumb or finger remains visible for some time as a 'dimple' in the tissue.

Initially this lymphoedema may reduce during the night, one of the reasons why it can sometimes be difficult to distinguish the first stage of lymphoedema from oedemas with another cause.

<u>Second stage</u>
As the lymphoedema increases further, more fluid accumulates in the interstitium causing the tissue to begin to fibrose. The pressure in the lymphatic system also increases, causing the vessel walls of the lymphangions to begin to fibrose. The transport capacity is further reduced as a result.
The tissue becomes harder and the pitting oedema from the first stage develops into non-pitting oedema. Stemmer's test is positive (see § 3.4.4). There is an increased susceptibility to infections.

The second stage is called 'spontaneous irreversible', there is no endogenous mechanism that can counteract this process. With adequate treatment a volume reduction may be achieved, but often at this stage irreparable tissue damage has already occurred.

Third stage

If the lymphoedema increases further this will lead to further tissue damage. The fibrotic tissue becomes even harder and affects more structures, such as arteries and veins. Due to the fibrosis nerve fibres may come under pressure and be damaged.
Skin deformities such as hyperkeratosis, cysts, fistulas and papillomas occur. Infections often occur.
This stage is also called 'lymphatic elephantiasis'. With adequate treatment an improvement can be achieved, but the tissue damage is permanent.

3.4.4 Identification of lymphoedema

The distinction of different forms of oedema can in practice be difficult and must be carried out by trained specialists. The treatment of both primary and secondary lymphoedema must also be carried out by specially trained oedema therapists.

As already previously stated, lymphoedema in practice occurs relatively frequently. Unfortunately lymphoedema is still always poorly identified and recognised. Therapists therefore have a considerable chance of being faced in their practice with people suffering from undiagnosed and therefore un-treated lymphoedema.

A very simple test can be carried out that gives almost 100% certainty of the presence of lymphoedema, namely Stemmer's sign. Stemmer's sign is positive if a thickened skin fold is present on the dorsal side of the second toe.

In lymphoedema the skin is thickened because of the fibrotic tissue, which means it is more difficult or even impossible to take hold of a skin fold in the toe. Because other forms of oedema do not cause fluid accumulation in the feet or toes, while this is true for lymphoedema, a positive Stemmer's sign is seen as virtual proof of the presence of lymphoedema.

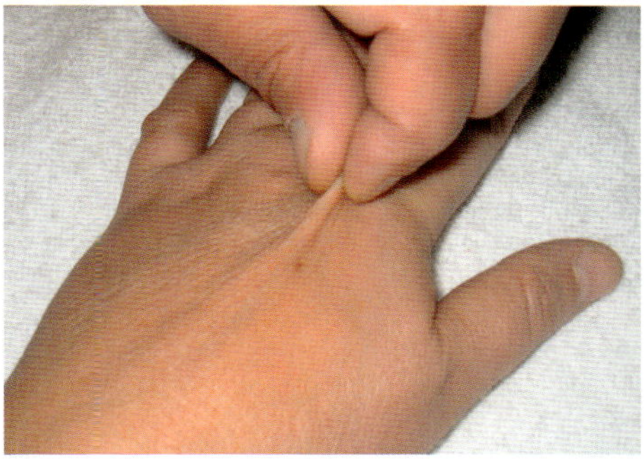

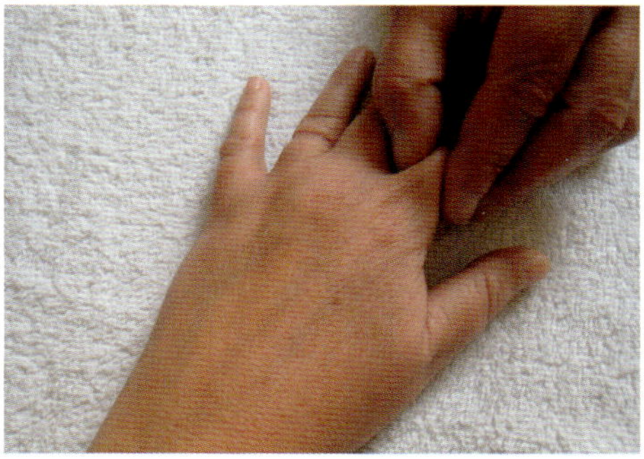

Positive Stemmer's sign.

Other forms of oedema do not occur in the upper extremities, while lymphoedema may occur there. Stemmer's sign can therefore also be used in the fingers to detect the presence of an arm lymphoedema. In the upper extremity Stemmer's sign is however of less value for early diagnosis.

According to the literature Stemmer's sign is never false positive. The test can however be false negative. The presence of lymphoedema cannot therefore be excluded if Stemmer's sign is negative.

If a positive Stemmer's sign is found, the client must be sent to a specialist therapist. In such a case it must be strongly advised not to start lymph taping or other therapies.

3.5 Other forms of oedema

In addition to lymphoedema, various other forms of oedema occur. In this paragraph venous oedema and lipoedema are discussed. Apart from these disorders that can be distinguished, in practice many mixed forms also occur, where the volume increase present is caused by different components.

3.5.1 Lipoedema and lipo-lymphoedema

Lipoedema is a symmetrically occurring, chronic condition, arising almost exclusively in women.
It is characterised by a symmetrical volume increase of the legs, usually from the pelvic brim to the ankles. The feet remain slim. If the lipoedema also occurs in the arms, the hands also remain slim.
Another noticeable feature is that lipoedema is tender, unlike lymphoedema. A third symptom is the rapidly occurring haematomas due to bleeding in the subcutaneous fatty tissue.

In lipoedema fat cells are pushed out of the subcutis into the dermis. Each fat cell has its own blood capillary, but there are no lymph capillaries between the fat cells. As a result a much greater distance has to be bridged before the pre-lymph between the fat cells can be absorbed by the lymphatic system.

Földi et al. describes how in lipoedema the characteristic changes occur due to microangiopathy between the fat cells. This microangiopathy consists of an increased fragility of the capillaries, which causes the rapidly occurring haematomas. At the same time there is an increased permeability, as a result of which more protein-rich fluid accumulates between the cells. The accumulation of more protein-rich fluid, together with the increased distance to the initial lymph vessels, makes the drainage of pre-lymph more difficult.

In the case of lipoedema abnormalities in the lymph vessels are also described, which reduce the functionality of these drainage vessels. The absorption of pre-lymph is made difficult, as is the transport of lymph.

In a progressing process a lipo-lymphoedema develops. The volume increase is then also seen in the feet and possibly the hands, Stemmer's sign is positive in this phase.

According to Földi lipoedema occurs very frequently, namely in 11% of women. In men lipoedema is rare and in these cases is associated with serious hormonal disorders or liver function disorders.

Lipoedema is often wrongly diagnosed as bilateral primary lymphoedema or as morbid obesity. The local fatty tissue in lipoedema does not disappear due to diet nor due to sport (see also § 3.4.1).

3.5.2 Venous oedema and phlebolymphoedema

Chronic venous insufficiency is a commonly occurring condition, over 12% of the adult population are affected by it. The main cause is formed by dysfunctional valves in the venous system, which causes a reflux of the venous blood. Venous oedema can be further caused by an obstruction in the veins (for example thrombosis) or by the absence of the supporting muscle pump (for example in case of paresis).

One of the earliest symptoms of chronic venous insufficiency is the occurrence of venous oedema. This is a pitting oedema that develops in the course of the day mainly around the ankles. During the night this oedema goes down again. Stemmer's sign is negative.

The increased venous pressure results in increased filtration. The lymphatic load therefore increases. Ultimately compensation via the lymphatic system will fail, which causes phlebolymphoedema. This is a dynamic insufficiency, the treatment is therefore not aimed at increasing the transport capacity. In other words, venous oedema is not an indication for lymph taping. The target for these forms of oedema must lie in the venous insufficiency.

4. Lymph taping

4.1 Introduction

The treatment of lymphoedema with lymph taping has been used increasingly since the beginning of this century. Compared with more conventional treatments, lymph taping also offers many benefits.

The use of compression therapy is however extensively documented and substantiated, where the substantiation for lymph taping as a relatively new treatment method still leaves a lot to be desired. The results obtained with lymph taping have ensured that there is a lot of national and international interest in it at present.

There are already a growing number of publications about lymph taping and in view of the number of international initiatives for scientific research into this subject, it may be expected that the quantity and the quality of publications will increase considerably in the years to come. It seems realistic to assume that this will further increase the theoretical substantiation of this method.

4.2 Effects of lymph taping

To be able to understand why lymph taping works, both knowledge of the specific properties of the material and anatomical and physiological knowledge of the lymphatic system is necessary.

The elastic CureTape is applied over the stretched skin, where the tape itself is not additionally stretched. When the stretched skin returns to the normal position, convolutions are created in the skin. The epidermis is slightly lifted, creating some space in the dermis. Here, in the interstitium of the dermis, is where most initial lymph vessels are located.

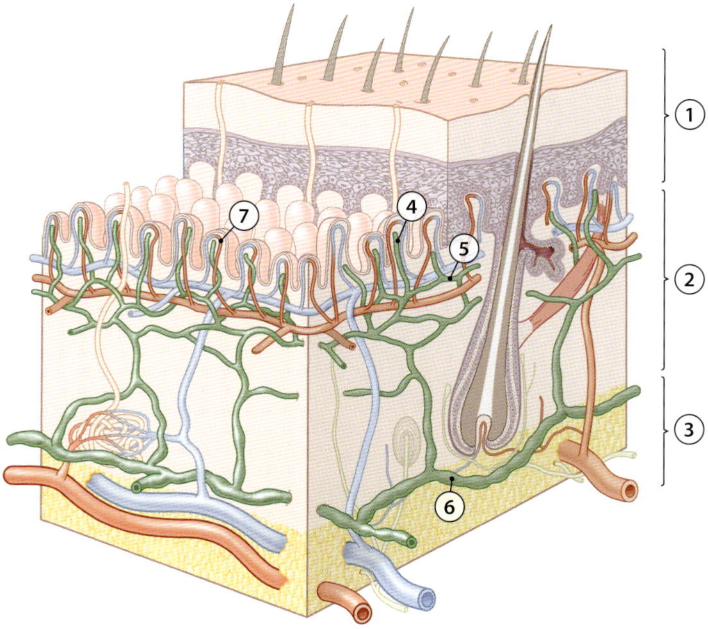

1. Epidermis
2. Dermis
3. Subcutis
4. Initial lymph vessels
5. Precollectors
6. Collectors
7. Microcirculation

Because the pressure under the tape is lower than in a skin region without tape, and water will move to the region with lower pressure, the free fluid in the interstitium will be 'sucked up' by the tape. During movement the convolutions created by the tape, will constantly increase and decrease. This can be thought of as a sort of micro massage effect.

Anatomically it is the initial lymph vessels and to a small extent the precollectors that absorb pre-lymph from the interstitium. Under normal circumstances the initial lymph vessels open when the pressure in the interstitium increases. However, if the pressure becomes too high, the initial lymph vessels will tend to be closed. The space under the tape causes a pressure reduction, so the initial lymph vessels can also absorb pre-lymph from the interstitium more easily.

The first stage of lymph transport in the precollectors also takes place due to pressure differences, certainly at points where this transport is not yet supported by valves or smooth muscle tissue.

In lymph taping, narrow strips of tape are applied with regular spaces between them. Under the narrow tape strips the pressure is lower than in the space between the tape strips. The complete lymph taping therefore creates an area with lots of pressure differences, which stimulates the absorption of pre-lymph and the first stage of lymph transport.

The lymph tape strips are applied here such that the tape can work in the optimum way possible as a conductor of fluid droplets. The anatomical substrate of a strip of lymph tape as a fluid conductor can be found in the prelymphatic channels that run along elastic fibrils. These elastic connective tissue fibres also have a function in conducting the free fluid.

The free fluid in the interstitium, the pre-lymph, will have to be absorbed somewhere by the lymphatic system so that it can actually be drained. The absorption of pre-lymph will occur at a place where this is also possible, in other words, where the pressure within the initial lymph vessels and the precollectors makes this possible. In other words: because the tape strips can function as a fluid conductor, the reabsorption area is increased.

From the initial lymph vessels and precollectors, the lymph must then flow to collectors to be drained further to central. If the pressure within the local collector is too high because the system is overloaded, the drainage to the local collector will not succeed.

Because both the initial lymph vessels and the precollectors form a network with one another, it will be possible for the lymph within this network to flow to a place where the pressure in the lymphatic system is lower and where there are drainage possibilities via the local collector.

The network of initial lymph vessels and the network of precollectors both lie just under the epidermis, in the layer of the dermis. This is the layer of tissue where tape can exert an effect. The collectors are located a little deeper, in the hypodermis, where in fact the tape cannot be expected to have a direct effect.

Because the pressure under the tape strips is lower, the lymph will also flow more easily under the tape strips, within the network of initial lymph vessels and within the network of precollectors, to an area where the pressure within the lymphatic system is lower. Here the lymph can flow further on to a collector.

To sum up:

1. Under the tape there is a lower pressure, which can 'suck up' free fluid;
2. Due to the lower pressure under the tape initial lymph vessels more easily absorb pre-lymph;
3. During exercise the changing convolutions present create a micro massage effect;
4. Pressure differences under the tape and in the space between the tape stimulate transport;
5. The tape strips can act as a conductor for the free fluid in the interstitium;
6. With the conducting tape strips the reabsorption area is increased;
7. Due to the lower pressure under the tape strips the transport of lymph within the networks of initial lymph vessels and precollectors is facilitated.

Lymph taping works as long as it sits on the skin. The tape therefore achieves a long term effect, similar to the effects of manual lymph drainage.

During manual lymph drainage however work can also be done in the deeper layers of tissue, while the lymph tape has its effect in the surface layer. Lymph taping in primary and secondary lymphoedema must therefore be seen as an adjunct to treatment with manual lymph drainage. In case of a temporarily overloaded, but in principle healthy lymphatic system, lymph taping may suffice as a treatment.

**With thanks to Dimitri Reder, who by his critical questions has contributed enormously to this paragraph.*

4.3 Lymph taping compared with manual lymph drainage

In the case of manual lymph drainage surface and deep massage is alternated. In the case of surface massage a number of objectives are aimed for. The stretching of the skin stimulates the absorption of pre-lymph by the initial lymph vessels. The stretching of the skin causes stretching of the anchor filaments, so the initial lymph vessels open more easily and absorb pre-lymph.
This is alternated with slight pressure in the direction of flow to promote transport. The alternating pressure reduction due to stretching of the skin and the slight pressure increase in the direction of flow supports lymph transport.
The similarities between the effects of lymph taping and the action of manual lymph drainage seem clear here. Both methods use pressure reduction, pressure changes and the emphasis of pressure differences to stimulate the surface lymphatic system.
In the case of manual lymph drainage there is a slight emphasis in the direction of lymph flow. In the case of lymph taping this happens insofar as the elastic tape is applied from the area to which the lymph must be transported. Then the strip of lymph tape is applied towards the oedema area. The elastic properties of the material provide a stimulus towards the first point positioned, the direction of action is the opposite to the tape direction.
During manual lymph drainage a further effect can also be exerted on slightly deeper collectors, which increases the lymphangion motor function. With deeper massage the lymph nodes can also be treated. Both factors can further promote lymph transport.

The effect of lymph taping is in the more surface layer, on the level of the initial lymph vessels and precollectors. The slightly deeper collectors and lymph nodes are not directly affected. Particularly in primary and secondary lymphoedema lymph taping therefore supplements treatment with manual lymph drainage. In the case of a primary or secondary lymphoedema, treatment with lymph taping should properly be performed by a specialist oedema therapist.

4.4 Lymph taping versus compression therapy

When treating lymphoedema it is usual following manual lymph drainage to apply compression in the form of bandages or compression stockings. The main objective here is also to maintain the benefit obtained during manual lymph drainage.

The pressure of stockings or bandages ensures an increased tissue pressure in the interstitium, which can increase (venous) reabsorption, while the capillary filtration of fluid is reduced.

Fluid or lymph that is absorbed in the venous system or in the lymphatic system will due to the pressure increase more readily flow in a direction where a lower pressure prevails, in this case to proximal.

In case of venous insufficiency, where the valve system is no longer working to the optimum, compression is used to reduce the diameter of the vessels so that the valve system is more functional again. It is assumed that this mechanism could also work for collectors with an insufficient valve system.

The use of compression therapy is theoretically well substantiated. In scientific studies into compression therapy there is however often no real control group because of the ethical consequences. Compression therapy clearly has a positive effect in case of lymphoedema. The empirical proof is overwhelming.

But for the person being treated with compression therapy, there are considerable consequences. Compression with bandages or stockings causes much discomfort and feels particularly unpleasant. During hotter and more oppressive weather conditions the discomfort from compression increases even more.

As already stated in the previous paragraph, lymph taping in primary and secondary lymphoedema is also used following treatment with manual lymph drainage. The purpose of lymph taping is however not only to maintain the effect of manual lymph drainage, the purpose of lymph taping is to stimulate a further absorption and drainage of lymph.

Lymph taping is however used following manual treatment. Treatment with manual lymph drainage is rather more intensive than treatment with tape, but even more importantly, during manual lymph drainage the experienced oedema therapist can also determine what anastomoses can be used for effective tape treatment.

Clients who have personally experienced what compression therapy involves virtually without exception experience treatment with lymph taping as an enormous relief. The tape is hardly felt at all and does not hinder them in their daily activities.

Chronic lymphoedema, as in the case of primary and secondary lymphoedema, has a considerable impact on various aspects of life. When stressful compression therapy is replaced by much better tolerated lymph taping, this means a considerable improvement in the quality of life.

4.5 Misunderstandings about lymph taping

4.5.1 Introduction

There are two fairly persistent misunderstandings about lymph taping, that both affect the choices made within treatment. In an attempt to dispel these misunderstandings, they are both described separately here.
The first problem concerns the question of whether it is necessary to respect the watershed with the lymph tape strips. The second problem is about the efficacy of lymph taping in case of lymphoedema in the lower extremities.
The third subject in this chapter concerns the question of whether the location of lymph node stations affects the starting point of the lymph tapes.

4.5.2 The effect of the watershed

A frequently heard comment is that the lymph tape strips should not extend beyond the watershed. A brief reminder of relevant anatomical aspects can provide clarification here.
As described in § 4.2, the action of lymph tapes should be sought in the surface layer of the tissue, at the level of prelymphatic channels, initial lymph vessels and precollectors. The prelymphatic channels do not respect the watershed (see § 2.2), and both the initial lymph vessels and precollectors form a network where lymph drainage is possible in all flow directions.

The initial lymph vessels together form overlapping skin areas, through which lymph can be drained in different directions. Precollectors that drain together to one collector, together form a skin zone. The skin zones are connected to one another by the overlapping skin areas, so that on this level too drainage is possible in all directions. (See § 2.3.1)

The watershed only occurs at the slightly deeper level of the collectors. Because during manual lymph drainage work can also be done in this slightly deeper layer the watershed is therefore important during manual treatment.

Lymph taping does however work on the more surface level of the initial lymph vessels and precollectors. The watershed therefore in no way has to affect the location of the lymph tape strips.

The view that lymph tape strips should respect the watershed is therefore wrong.

4.5.3 Lymph taping for the lower extremities

The view is expressed with some regularity that lymph taping is not, or in any case is less, effective for lymphoedema in the legs. A number of comments can be made about this.

As long as this involves the treatment of lymphoedema, the problem is similar to the problem found in other parts of the body. The system to be influenced is also similar. Anatomically and physiologically there is therefore no reason to assume that the efficacy of the lymph tapes in the lower extremities should be any different compared for example with the upper extremities.

Lymphoedema in the lower extremities may occur in three different situations. The first situation in principle involves a healthily functioning lymphatic system, which is temporarily overloaded. Often this will be even more local, as a result of a trauma or surgical procedure.

The lymph tape in that case conducts lymph to an area that has more absorption capacity. The lymphatic system is healthy, and absorption in another area will not cause any problems.

The second situation involves secondary lymphoedema that has arisen because there has been damage to the lymphatic system, which has reduced the drainage capacity. Here too it is possible to use lymph taping to conduct the lymph to an area where the absorption and drainage capacity is still intact. The efficacy is comparable with the efficacy of lymph taping for secondary lymphoedema in the upper extremities.

In primary lymphoedema the biggest problem often arises in the lower extremities, the third situation. In this situation there are not enough lymph vessels, or the lymph vessels are not functioning sufficiently. The operating principles of lymph taping do however remain the same. The lymph is conducted via the surface system to an area with more absorption capacity. Because lymph taping acts in the surface system, lymph taping is effective even if the collectors are not functioning (the valves do not close or not sufficiently). Observations from practice fully concur with this.

Apart from lymphoedema, venous oedema may also be present in the lower extremities. In that case the venous drainage is insufficient, usually because the valves in the veins no longer close properly. The majority of the fluid that has to be drained from the interstitium is absorbed into the venous system. Even a healthily functioning lymphatic system will not be able to compensate sufficiently for the failure of the venous system. In case of venous oedema the compression from outside is necessary to reduce the diameter of the venous vessels, so that the venous drainage can improve again. Venous oedema is therefore not an indication for the use of lymph taping.

In practice mixed venous-lymphoedema regularly occurs. The total volume increase in the legs may partly be caused by lymphoedema, and partly by venous oedema. In that case the efficacy of lymph taping will depend on the proportion of the lymph component with respect to the venous component. The greater the share of venous oedema, the less effective lymph taping will be.

In the case of lipoedema or lipo-lymphoedema, lymph taping also has an added value in the treatment. Even in these situations with lymph taping the free fluid in the interstitium can be conducted to an area where more lymph absorption and transport is possible.

Lymph taping for the lower extremities is exactly as effective as in other parts of the body, at least as long as this involves the treatment of lymphoedema.

4.5.4 Taping from a lymph node station?

In the development of the lymph taping technique, the base of a lymph tape was always positioned by a lymph node station. The thought behind this was that the lymph could then be transported in most optimum way in the direction of the central lymph node stations.

Since it should be concluded that the action of lymph tape mainly takes place at the level of the initial lymph vessels and precollectors, where the absorption and first stage of the transport take place, it does not seem logical for lymph tape to always be applied from a lymph node station. After all the lymph nodes themselves are not able to absorb lymph.

Another important idea about the action of lymph tape, concerns the possibility of using tape strips to conduct free fluid to a place where there are better possibilities of fluid being absorbed. The longer strips used for this, provide a longer pathway and hence more possibilities for the absorption of lymph into the lymphatic system. From this reasoning it may then be sensible to start the lymph tape level with a lymph node station, to make optimum use of the longer distance and hence the increased reabsorption area.

4.6 Lymph taping, the technique

4.6.1 Stretch in the tape

Lymph taping is in principle a standard technique. When applying lymph tape the skin is therefore stretched and the tape strips are positioned without additional stretching, but maintaining 10% pretensioning.

If it is not possible to stretch the skin sufficiently, this can be compensated for by stretching the skin by hand in the direction of the base of the lymph strip.

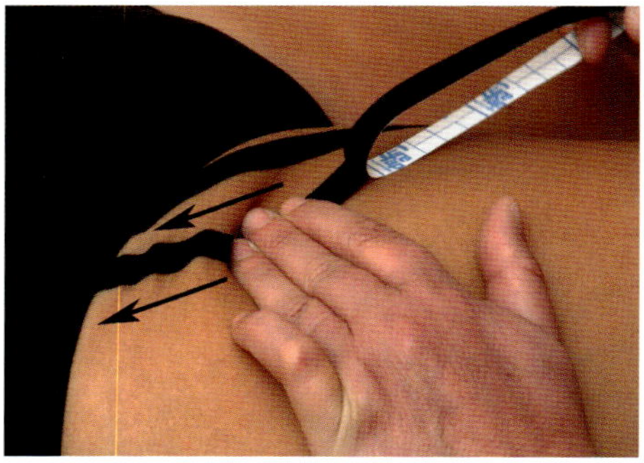

Stretching the skin by hand.

When treating fibroses or adhering scars it is recommended that slightly more stretch is incorporated in the tape, see for this § 5.7.

4.6.2 Width of the tape strips

For lymph taping narrow strips of tape are used. The narrower the strips that are used, the more effective the lymph tape treatment will be. The disadvantage of strips that are too narrow is that the tape construction becomes more delicate and will come loose more quickly. Furthermore applying strips of tape that are too narrow is very time-consuming, certainly if a large area has to be treated.

If wider lymph strips are used, then there is a loss of efficacy, but the tape construction does remain in place better. There is an (arbitrary) turning point at which the tape strips are too wide to still produce sufficient effect. Based on observations in practice, the conclusion has been drawn that lymph tape strips of 2½ cm wide are in fact too wide to achieve a good treatment result.

The choice of the ultimate width of the tape strips may partly depend on the part of the body being taped and the size of the area to be treated. On the face narrow strips will tend to be used, for example 0.8 cm wide (= 5 cm wide tape cut into 6 strips). For a complete leg the choice of 1.6 cm wide tape (= 5 cm wide tape cut into 3 strips) may offer advantages.

4.6.3 Direction of the tape strips

Because the direction of action of the tape is the opposite to the tape direction, the base of a lymph tape is always located in the area to which the lymph must be transported. The anchor of the lymph strip comes in the area where the lymphatic pressure is too high.

The lymphatic system is a draining system from the periphery to central. In the extremities lymph tape is therefore applied from central to peripheral. The only exception to this is often (but not always!) for taping on the back of the hand. On the back of the hand lymph tape is usually more effective if the tape is applied from distal to proximal (see also § 5.4.8).

4.6.4 Length of the lymph strips

The lymph strips are applied from the target area to the problem area. The aim is to reduce the pressure of fluid in the problem area as far as possible. For this reason the lymph strips therefore end proximal from the problem area or in the problem area.

The strips do not end peripheral from the problem area. Should however the strips end peripheral from the problem area, then the peripheral section of the tape will stimulate the transport of fluid to the problem area. This is always undesirable.

If taping is carried out proximal from the problem area, the lymphatic pressure in this region will be lower. Because fluid tends to move in the direction where the pressure is lower, a proximal lymph tape will therefore exert a sucking action on the fluid in the problem area.

By working proximal from the problem area with longer strips, such as for an anastomosis tape, the conducting function of the tape is used. Due to the longer distance the reabsorption area increases which can increase the result.

4.6.5 Space between the strips

It is possible to work with more or less space between the tape strips. By using less space between the lymph strips, the total lymph tape construction can be more intensive. More space between the strips gives a slightly less intensive tape construction.

If the space between the strips is too narrow or the strips even lie up against one another, then the ultimate result is comparable to the effect of a wider tape strip. This will reduce the treatment result.

In the case of an intensive lymph tape construction the space between the strips can be roughly as wide as the width of the lymph strip.

4.6.6 Combined techniques

For various indications it is possible and sensible in addition to lymph tape to also use other techniques, for example to support muscle or ligament structures.

If working with combinations of tape techniques, the lymph tapes must ALWAYS be applied FIRST. This maintains the pressure differences created, while these pressure differences may be reduced or disappear if the order is reversed.
The other tape techniques can then be chosen according to the treatment priority.

4.7 Choices in tape forms

In the relatively short history of lymph taping, there has been a constant search for tape forms that can improve the result further. The different lymph tape forms have their own characteristics and corresponding advantages and disadvantages.

4.7.1 Fan shape versus separate strips

For the fan shape, 5 cm wide tape or 7½ cm wide tape is cut into several narrow strips, which remain fixed to one another at the base.

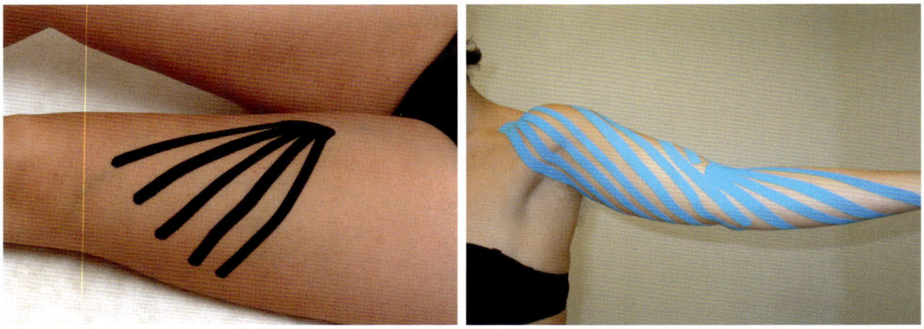

Photo left: fan-shaped tape local.
Photo right: fan-shaped tapes applied over the whole arm, from supraclavicular to the elbow and from the elbow to the wrist.

Initially these fan-shaped tapes were positioned from one lymph node station to the next lymph node station, where the lymph strips were applied in a spiral.

Advantage: the tape strips can be slightly shorter, which makes applying the tape easier.

Disadvantage: two disadvantages can be mentioned. In the first place the fact is that remarkably little tape irritation occurs in people who are treated with lymph taping. But if tape irritation does occur, then it is with the fan-shaped tapes and virtually without exception only under the base of the tape, that is where the lymph strips are fixed to one another.
The second disadvantage is that the tape strips must be applied spread out from the base. At the base it is therefore easy for folds to occur in the tape, which also cause skin irritation.

In the explanation of the action of lymph taping, it is stated that the tape strips can act as a conductor for the free fluid in the interstitium. If that is so, then a lot of fluid could be collected under the base of the tape with this fan-shaped tape. Furthermore this base was always placed level with a lymph node station, where the skin is often very sensitive. Both reasons can cause skin irritation to occur under the base of the tape.

By cutting right through the tape, separate strips are created that each have their own base and anchor. These separate strips can be placed as a whole from the target area to the problem area.

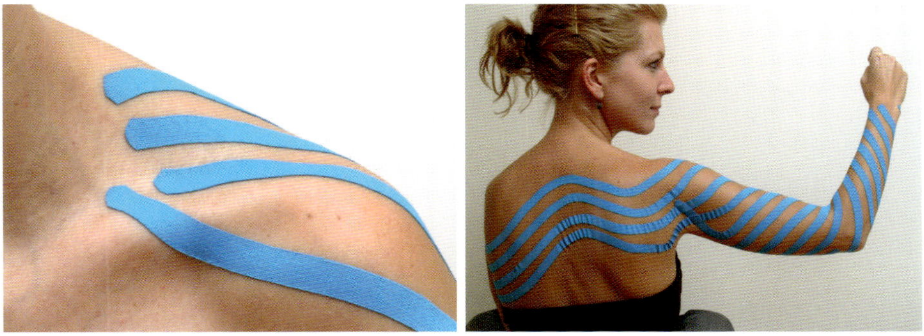

Separate strips of tape over the whole arm, the bases of the strips lie separate from one another supraclavicular.

Advantage: several advantages can be mentioned. The problem of skin irritation is greatly reduced in this way; the tape strips are applied without a break; much more flexibility is possible in forming the total tape construction; if necessary one tape strip can be removed from it without damaging the rest of the tape construction; the chance of folds in the tape at the base is greatly reduced.

Disadvantage: the application of the tape requires slightly more experience because of the length of the tape strips.

With this method one must ensure that the bases of the different tape strips are not applied in too concentrated a way, because then a similar situation arises as with a fan-shaped tape.

4.7.2 Spiral, anatomical or wavelike

Both fan-shaped tapes and lymph tapes composed of separate strips can be applied in three different ways.

1. Spiral
   With the spiral form the strips are applied round the arm or leg in an elongated spiral. The original thought behind this is that in this way the lymph vessels (collectors) are crossed at several heights, which can give a greater treatment result.
2. Anatomical
   With a more anatomically applied tape the strips largely follow the anatomical course of the collectors. This method arose from the thought that the watersheds should be respected.
3. Wavelike
   Here the lymph strips are laid down in a wavelike pattern. The idea is that the watershed can in this way be respected and that the wavelike shape could have a better conducting function.

The explanation of how lymph taping works is based on the effect that the tape has on the network of the initial lymph vessels and the network of precollectors. From this explanation it must be concluded that all these three forms can be equally effective. The arguments about the watershed and the course of the collectors, as described earlier in this chapter, are not important.

If there is a difference in the efficacy of these different forms of lymph tapes, that should be looked for in the function of the tape as a fluid conductor. The action of a spiral shaped tape where the spirals are applied too flat or too horizontal does in fact decrease.

One point to be borne in mind for the spiral shaped tape is therefore that the tape must be positioned in extended gradual spirals. If the tape is applied too horizontally, the conducting function is reduced.

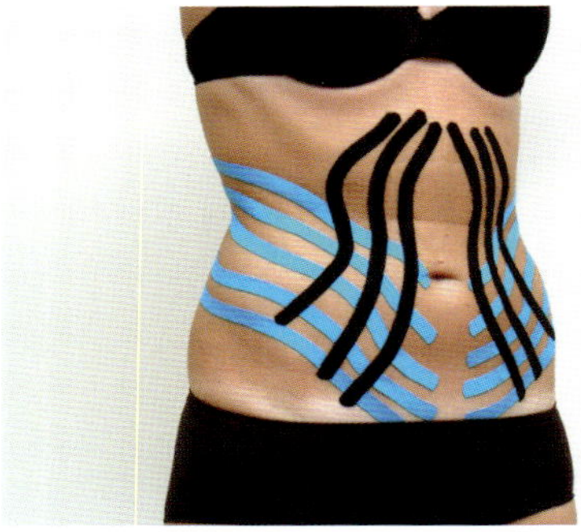
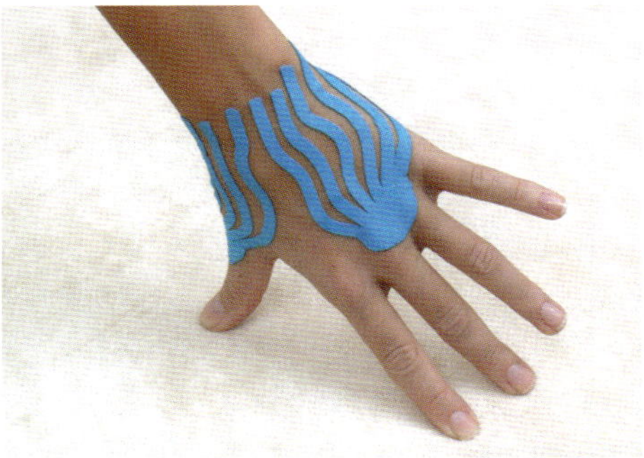

Photo left: lymph tape composed of separate strips; here a combination of spiral shaped strips and wavelike strips. Photo right: lymph tape in a fan shape, where the strips are applied in a wavelike fashion.

A spiral shaped tape exerts its action in the supply area of several collectors; a vertical ('anatomical') tape always exerts its action in the supply area of the same collector/collectors. This could mean that in the case of healthily and functionally laid out collectors the effect of a spiral shaped lymph tape is no, or hardly any, different from the effect of an anatomical lymph tape.
However where less functional collectors are involved, as in the case of primary lymphoedema, it may offer advantages that a spiral shaped tape exerts its action in the supply area of several collectors.

There is another point to be borne in mind in the case of lymph taping applied in a wavelike fashion. Allowance must be made for the fact that in the 'outer bend' there is automatically a little more stretch in the tape. At the same time in the 'inner bend' there is a risk of folds occurring in the tape. In places where folds are left in the tape, blistering or skin irritation may easily occur. Because any form of skin irritation may cause a greater lymphatic load, particularly when taping lymph problems, it is very important that this skin irritation cannot arise. The wavelike lymph tape must therefore be applied with small, gradual curves.

At present there are both therapists and those treated who consider one of these three tape forms to be more effective than the other forms. Whether this is in fact the case, will have to be proved by future research.

4.7.3 Parallel or crossed

In the case of an in principle healthily functioning lymphatic system, a local swelling or haematoma is often treated with a local grid shaped tape construction. With this grid tape small lymph strips are used, laid from two different directions.

Because the tape strips cross one another, small skin regions are covered by one layer of tape, by two layers of tape or remain free of tape. This causes a local increase in pressure differences, which is conducive to the absorption of lymph.

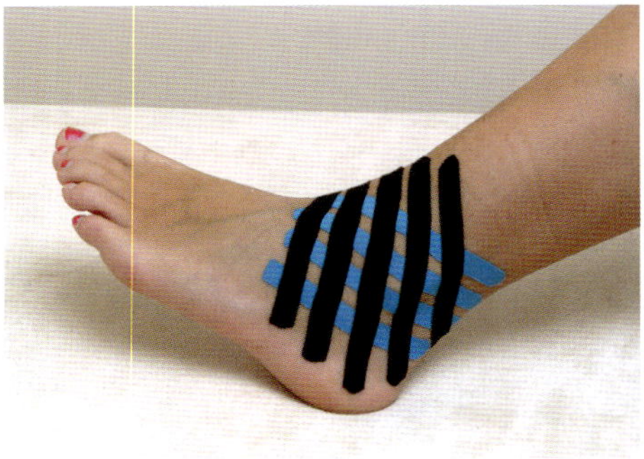

Local grid, short lymph tapes from proximal to distal, crossing in the area with swelling.

The same principle can be used for lymph taping for bigger areas, for example extremities with lymphoedema resulting from primary or secondary lymphoedema.

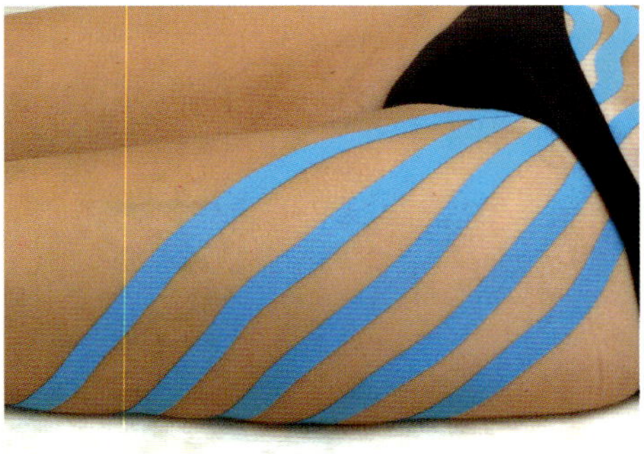

Parallel lymph taping.

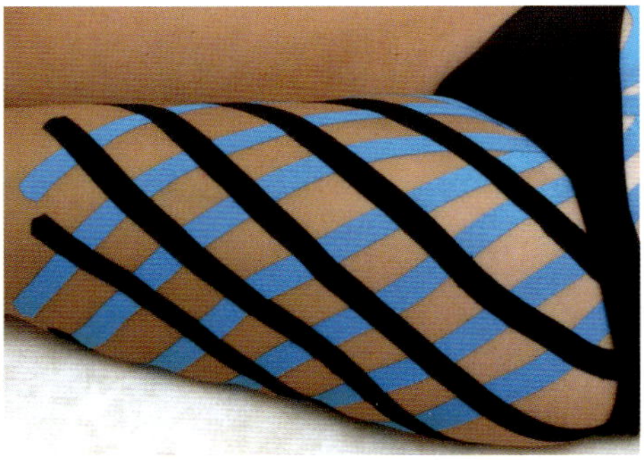

Crossed lymph taping.

Compared with parallel lymph taping, crossed lymph taping has an even more intensive action. In most cases this action is even too intensive. Crossed lymph taping is therefore only used for severe to very severe forms of oedema.

4.8 Treatment structure and treatment intensity

Particularly for the structure of treatment with lymph taping, it makes a difference whether the treatment is in a healthy and intact lymphatic system, or whether the treatment is for primary or secondary lymphoedema. These situations are therefore described in different paragraphs.

4.8.1 Structure and intensity in a healthy lymphatic system

Many situations are conceivable in which an in principle healthily functioning lymphatic system is still temporarily overloaded, or can use some extra support. As described in chapter 5, very different problems may be involved. For example swellings due to trauma, swellings due to overload, but also for example caused by colds or inflammations.

The body regulates this temporary overload, in other words, even without treatment the problem will in most cases disappear again of its own accord. Sometimes this happens too slowly, so complications may occur. For example the fibroses in the tissue that may occur as a result of a substantial haematoma. Furthermore the increased pressure in the tissue may hinder recovery. In all these cases lymph taping has its value as (part of the) treatment.

In general this temporary overload will be a local problem, for which local treatment may be enough. A local grid can then be applied with relatively short strips as described in § 5.7.1. This local treatment has a low intensity.

There may be various factors that affect the choice of more intensive treatment with lymph tape, such as:

- The severity of the problem;
- Underlying pathology (for example rheumatoid arthritis);
- Additional pathology (for example reflex dystrophy);
- Use of medication (for example blood-thinning medication);
- A combination with other injury.

It may be decided to apply more intensive lymph taping. In case of more intensive treatment longer lymph strips can be used from a drainage area located further away. Parallel strips can be used, or strips that cross one another. These methods differ mainly in treatment intensity.

Overall the structure in treatment intensity is rising from less to more intensive:

1. Local lymph strips, applied parallel (example: § 5.2.1);
2. Local lymph strips, applied crossed (example § 5.5.4);
3. Lymph strips from a drainage area located further away, applied parallel (example: § 5.3.4);
4. Local lymph strips, applied parallel combined with longer strips from a drainage area located further away which cross the local strips (example: § 5.4.5);
5. Parallel lymph strips from two different drainage areas located further away, crossing one another in the problem area (example: § 5.3.5);
6. Crossing lymph strips from a drainage area located further away (example: § 5.5.7).

Of course the treatment intensity may also be affected by varying the number of strips, or the space between the strips (see § 4.6.5).

For the first treatment based on the presenting situation a choice will be made in the treatment intensity. If this treatment has a good result, then for the follow-up treatment less intensive lymph taping is normally used.

4.8.2 Structure and intensity in primary or secondary lymphoedema

The treatment of primary or secondary lymphoedema always starts with manual lymph drainage and is therefore carried out by specialist oedema therapists. There is a specific treatment structure to manual lymph drainage. If manual lymph drainage is supplemented with lymph tape treatment, the lymph tape is adapted to the manual lymph drainage. In other words, the lymph tape is not applied further distal than the area which the therapist has treated during manual lymph drainage.

In case of fluid accumulation in the distal parts of the extremities, it is far from always necessary during manual lymph drainage to work entirely to distal. If the lymphatic pressure falls in the proximal area, the lymph flow into the distal area will automatically get going better. If it is enough only to drain in the proximal area, the lymph tape is also only applied in the proximal area.

Examination and manual treatment gives the therapist information about the severity of the problem, the sites with more or less severe problems and the alternative drainage paths that can be used. The ultimate lymph tape is based on this information. A choice must be made between the drainage areas that will be used, and the intensity of the tape treatment.

Increasing in treatment intensity, the following lymph tape constructions can be used:

1. Lymph strips from a drainage area located further away, applied parallel;
2. Local lymph strips, applied parallel combined with longer strips from one or more drainage areas located further away which cross the local strips;
3. Parallel lymph strips from one or more drainage areas located further away, crossing one another in the problem area;
4. Crossing lymph strips from one or more drainage areas located further away.

The treatment intensity can also be affected by varying the number of strips, or the space between the strips (see § 4.6.5). The different treatment examples are given in chapter 6 and chapter 7.

In view of the nature of the problems in primary or secondary lymphoedema, during manual lymph drainage work is often done to stimulate anastomoses. Manual treatment is however limited in time, so only one or two anastomoses can be worked on.

With lymph taping anastomoses can also be stimulated, where the work can be much more flexible and several possible anastomoses can be worked on at the same time. The lymph congestion will most readily be drained to an area with a lower lymphatic pressure. By stimulating several anastomoses at the same time, a much bigger possible spread is used, or, the reabsorption area thus correspondingly is increased.

5. Healthy lymphatic system with temporary overload

5.1 Introduction

A properly functioning lymphatic system can temporarily be subjected to an extra heavy load or even overloaded. Although this temporary overload generally also disappears again without treatment, many reasons can be given for still treating it with lymph taping.

The first reason that can be given is that the temporary overload can cause complications, such as fibroses. Secondly the local volume increase can cause pain due to the increased pressure in the tissue. This pain is reduced under the effect of lymph taping. Furthermore the fact is that tissue irritation causes swelling, but this swelling may cause further tissue irritation. The application of lymph taping can break this vicious circle.

This chapter deals with a variety of possibilities and indications. Case reports from practice alternate here with examples demonstrated with a photo model.

In a properly functioning lymphatic system treatment with lymph taping does not have to be preceded by manual lymph drainage. The lymph tape can if necessary be combined with other tape techniques, such as orthopaedic tapes.

Also in a healthily functioning lymphatic system the points to be borne in mind described in chapter 4 apply and must be taken into account if lymph taping is used.

5.2 Head and face

The lymphatic system in the face drains via the angle of mandible to supraclavicular, both on the left and on the right side. Lymph taping cannot be applied spirally here. Straight strips or a wavelike tape with gradual curves are used.

5.2.1. Sinusitis

In case of a (frontal) sinusitis 3 to 4 lymph strips can be applied to the left and right side of the face from the angle of mandible to just under the cheekbone.

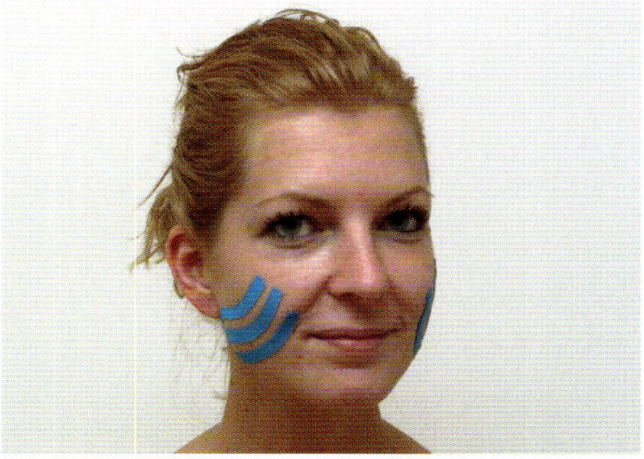

Lymph strips from the angle of mandible to the cheekbone in a gradual wave.
Width of the tape strips: here ± 0.8 cm (5 cm wide tape cut into 6 strips).

The tape strips are positioned proximal from the problem area. The drainage is stimulated under the tape strips, creating a lower pressure in the proximal area. As a result the lymphatic load in the problem area will move to the region with a lower pressure. The problem area is in this way relieved.

If there is also pressure in the neck area, or if the pressure in the neck area is uncomfortably increased by this, it may be decided to work with longer lymph strips, for example from supraclavicular. This increases the possibilities for absorption and transport of fluid.

The neck area is an extremely sensitive skin area, where irritation can very quickly arise if due to an incorrect technique the lymph strips are applied with too much stretch.

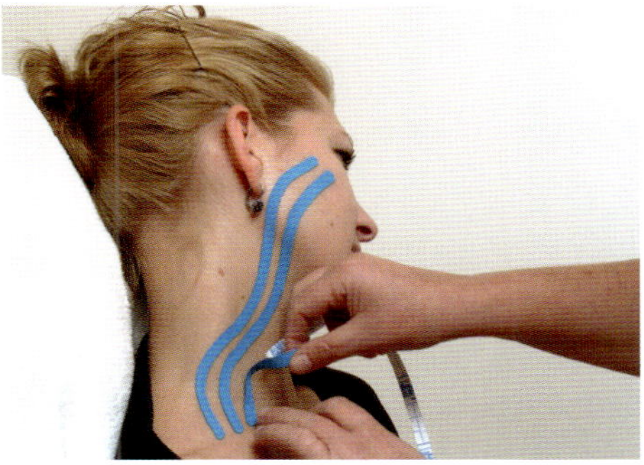

Lymph strips from supraclavicular to the cheekbone in a gradual wave.
Width of the tape strips: here ± 0.8 cm (5 cm wide tape cut into 6 strips).

The effect of this tape can be further intensified by positioning a 2 to 3 cm wide tape over the bridge of the nose, from the point of the nose to the root of the nose. Due to the lifting effect of the tape breathing through the nose remains easier as a result. This tape is also applied without extra stretch in the tape.

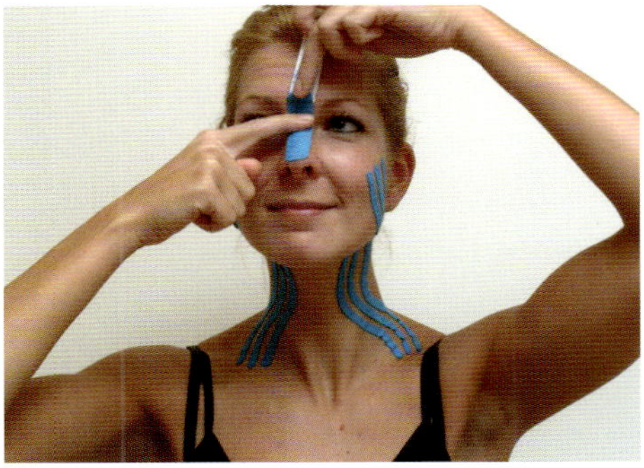

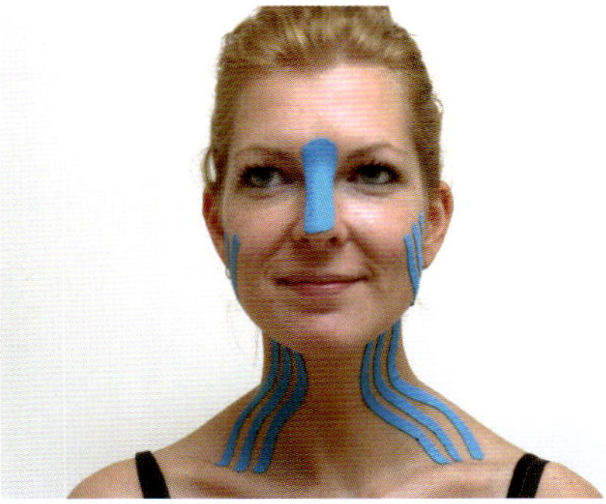

Tape on the bridge of the nose from the point of the nose to the root of the nose.
Width of the tape: 2 to 2 ½ cm.

This latter tape can also be used in case of snoring, where the snoring is caused by reduced fluid drainage.

5.2.2 Irritation or inflammations in the jaw area

In case of inflammations in the jaw area the pain can be alleviated by reducing the pressure in the inflammation area with lymph tape. Of course this tape construction is symptomatic and cannot be seen as the solution to the problem.

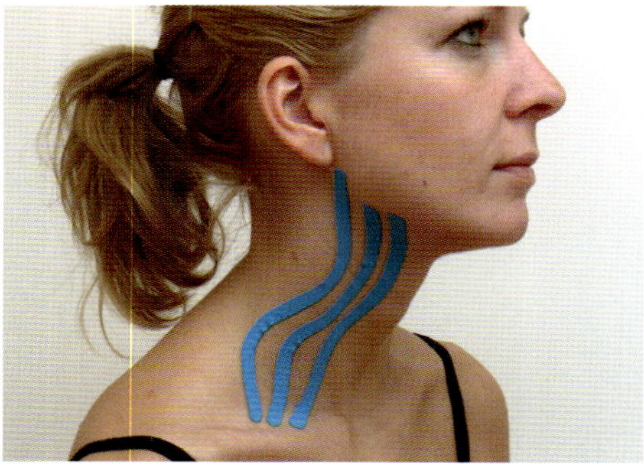

Lymph strips positioned from supraclavicular to the jaw line in a gradual wave.
Width of the tape strips: here ± 0.8 cm (5 cm wide tape cut into 6 strips).

Taping is carried out unilaterally to the side of the problem area, from supraclavicular to just under the jaw line. If the inflammation area is more central or even bilateral, the tape is applied to both sides.

The swelling after maxillary surgery or after a visit to the dentist can be treated with the same tape construction. If the tape is applied as quickly as possible after the procedure, in part it prevents swelling occurring. The pain after the procedure can in this way be reduced to a minimum.

5.2.3 Ear infections

In case of an ear infection the pressure in the problem area can be reduced by positioning three to four lymph strips from supraclavicular to under the ear. The tape is only applied to the side of the inflammation.

The strips are spread over the area just before, just under and just behind the start of the ear.

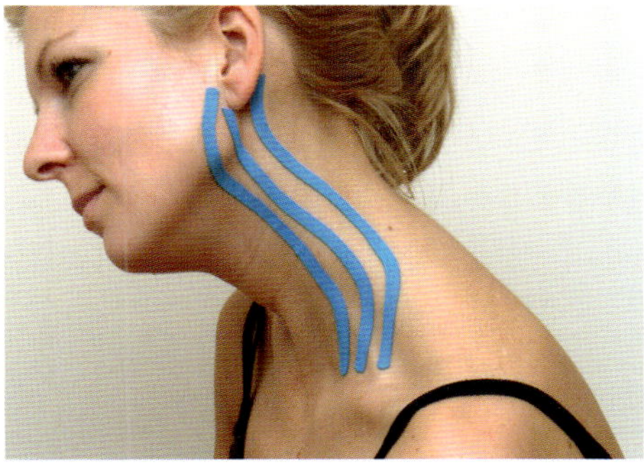

Lymph strips from supraclavicular to the underside of the ear, in a gradual wave.
Width of the tape strips: here ± 0.8 cm (5 cm wide tape cut into 6 strips).

The tape strips are positioned proximal from the problem area. The drainage under the tape strips is stimulated, creating a lower pressure in the proximal area. As a result the lymphatic load in the problem area will move to the region with a lower pressure.

This tape construction can in certain cases also be used in case of tinnitus.

5.2.4 Eyelid corrections or swelling around the eyes

In case of swelling around the eyes or a haematoma around the eyes such as for example occurs after eyelid corrections, lymph taping can be applied from the angle of mandible or from supraclavicular.

The tape strips are spread under the cheekbone edge and on the outside of the eye. The strips may not end in the soft part of the eye socket, because this causes too much irritation.

The tape construction from supraclavicular stimulates drainage of the swelling even more. An allowance must then be made for the sensitivity of the skin in the neck area, which can easily cause irritation in case of errors in technique.

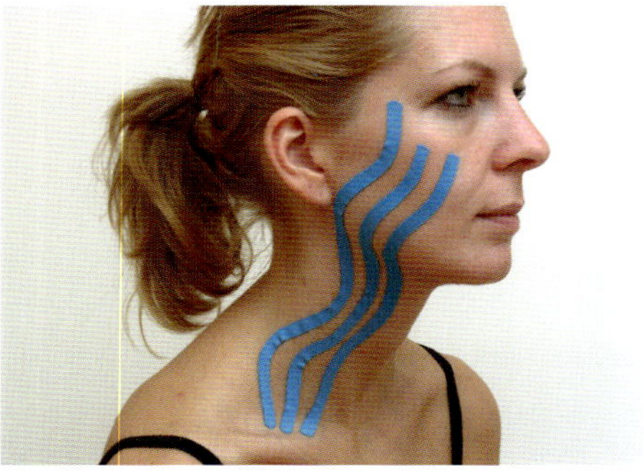

Lymph tape from supraclavicular to the cheekbone and the outside of the eye, in a gradual wave.
Width of the tape strips: here ± 0.8 cm (5 cm wide tape cut into 6 strips).

The tape strips are positioned proximal from the problem area. The drainage under the tape strips is stimulated, which creates a lower pressure in the proximal area. As a result the lymphatic load in the problem area will move to the region with a lower pressure.

5.2.5 Facial trauma

After a facial trauma in which the nose is bruised or broken, the following tape will have a very relieving action. Because taping and tape removal on a bruised or broken nose will be extremely painful, here too taping is carried out proximal from the problem area.

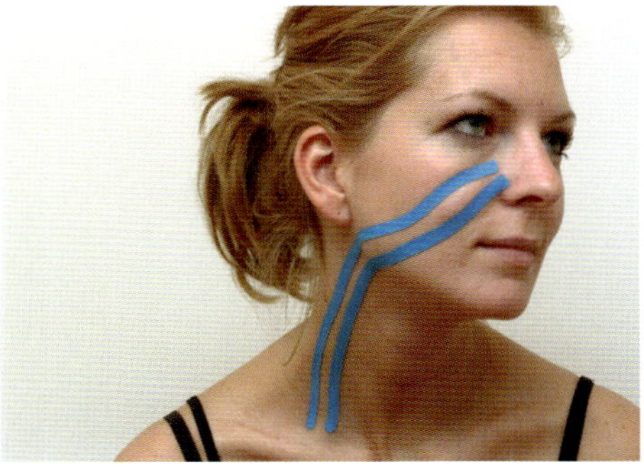

Lymph strips from supraclavicular to the side of the nose, in a gradual wave.
Width of the tape strips: here ± 0.8 cm (5 cm wide tape cut into 6 strips).

If the underside of the nose or the upper lip is also injured in the trauma, the above tape can be extended with a lymph strip to the upper lip.

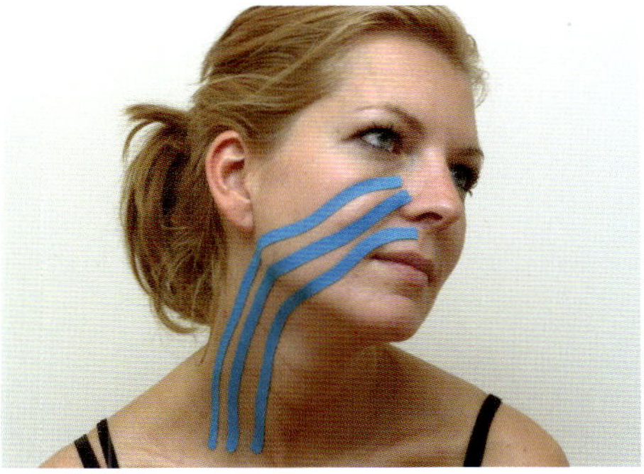

Lymph strips from supraclavicular to the side of nose and upper lip, in a gradual wave.
Width of the tape strips: here ± 0.8 cm (5 cm wide tape cut into 6 strips).

If the trauma has had a more considerable impact so that the lower lip is also swollen, the tape construction is further extended with a lymph strip to the lower lip.

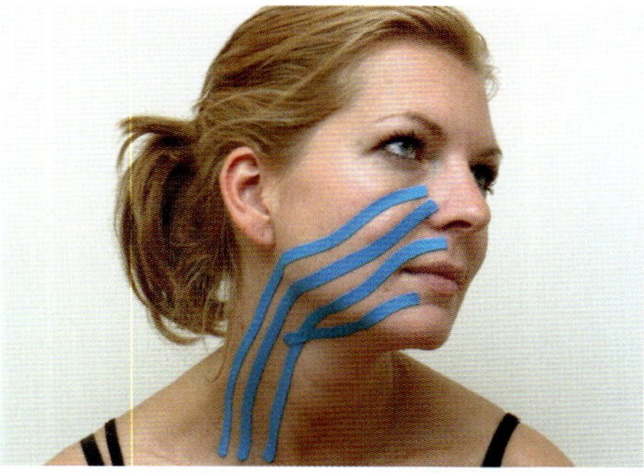

Lymph strips from supraclavicular to the side of nose, upper lip and lower lip.
Width of the tape strips: here ± 0.8 cm (5 cm wide tape cut into 6 strips).

For the lymph strip to the lower lip a branch is used here from the lymph strip in the direction of the upper lip.

If mainly swelling around the lips or of the mouth is involved, then the lymph strips are only applied to the problem area.

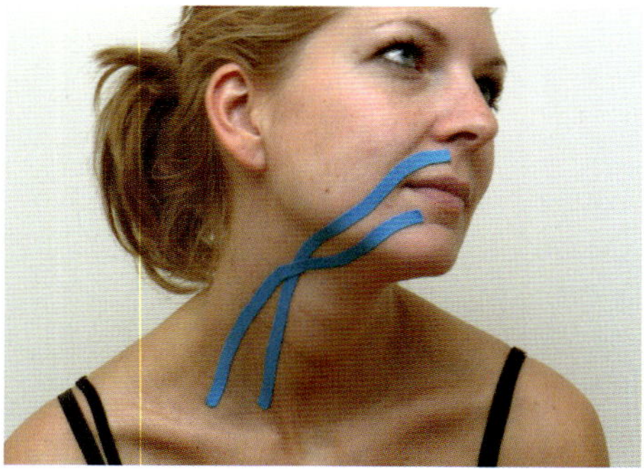

Lymph strips from supraclavicular to upper lip and lower lip.
Width of the tape strips: here ± 0.8 cm (5 cm wide tape cut into 6 strips).

The lymph strips in the figure cross over one another. That will not have an adverse effect on the action of the tape.
(cf: taping in case of haematomas, § 5.7).

5.3 Spine, back and abdomen

5.3.1 Cervical spine, case 8

Case description:

A hairdresser, 37 years, comes into the practice with pain symptoms in the right elbow. The GP's diagnosis is tennis elbow. Although in the examination it is noticed that the head is in anteroposition and a swelling is present around the cervico-thoracic area, the further examination of the cervical spine gives no reason to assume that the elbow symptoms are caused by the cervical spine. It is decided to carry out local treatment (see also: § 5.4.6).
During the third treatment it is found that the symptoms are diminishing, but that the level of symptoms remains higher than might be expected. Furthermore the symptoms appear to increase again immediately as soon as the local elbow tape is removed.
It is therefore decided to extend the treatment with lymph tape over the swelling in the cervico-thoracic transition area.

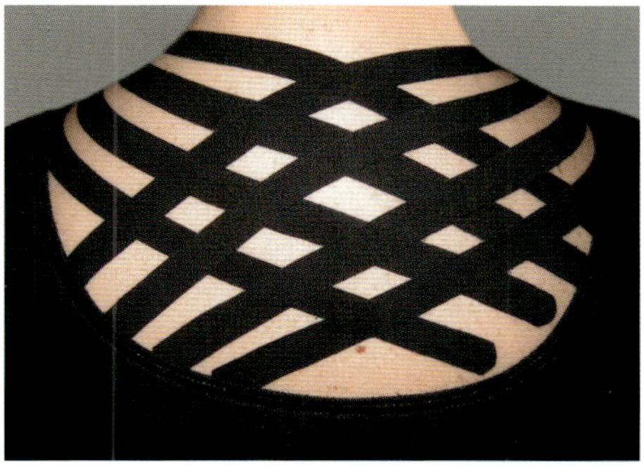

Bilateral lymph strips from supra-clavicular, crossing in the problem area.
Width of the tape strips: here ± 1.25 cm (5 cm wide tape cut into 4 strips).

By having the tape strips cross in the problem area, the emphasis of the treatment lies here. The local elbow treatment is further continued.
After this any treatment gives a clear but gradual improvement, a reduction in symptoms that also remains present when the tape is removed.
After 3 treatments where both local tape and cervical tape is used, the client is symptom free.

5.3.2 Whiplash, case 12

Case description:

A cleaning lady, 35 years, comes into the practice because of fibromyalgia. This diagnosis was made 15 years ago by the neurologist. She has a moderate physical capacity and describes an extensive symptom pattern where in particular the pain in the thoracic spine and around the cervico-thoracic area stands out.

In the examination no movement restrictions are found to be present. There is however a noticeable and ample swelling around the cervico-thoracic area and to a lesser extent a swelling around Th8/Th9. Furthermore many active trigger points are found to be present. Shoulders and head tend to anteroposition.

The treatment is started with a combination of limited lymph taping and orthopaedic tapes. The orthopaedic tapes are mainly aimed at correcting the posture. The lymph strips are positioned bilaterally from the armpit area to the CTJ area, where the strips cross over one another in the problem area.

The treatment gives a good result. The pain symptoms are greatly diminished, the client is sleeping better and uses considerably less medication. By the third treatment the biggest problem is a stiff and tense feeling in the neck which extends to the right shoulder and deltoid region.

It is decided to extend the treatment with the lymph tapes, but to omit the orthopaedic tapes.

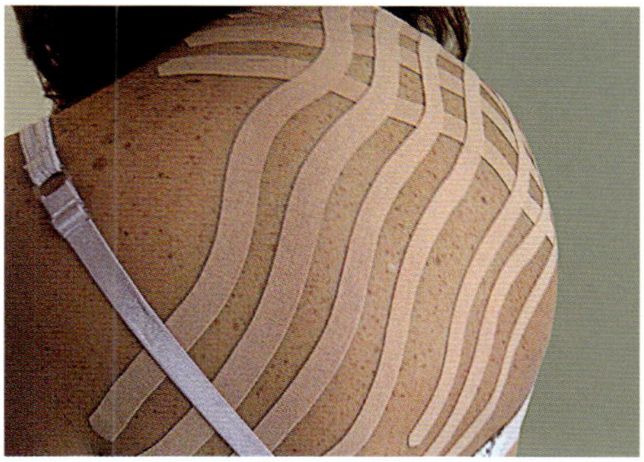

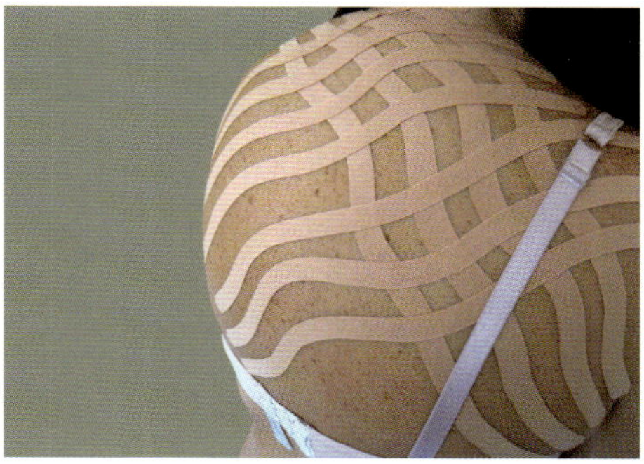

Bilateral lymph strips from the heterolateral axillary crossing into the CTJ area.
The lymph strips from the right armpit run to just into the left M. Trapezius area.
The lymph strips from the left armpit and lower from left heterolateral-paravertebral, end in the right M. Trapezius area and the top of the M. Deltoideus area.
Width of the tape strips: here ± 1.25 cm (5 cm wide tape cut into 4 strips).

This treatment is continued for a further three weeks with a frequency of 1 treatment per week. The intensity of the treatment is gradually reduced. By the sixth treatment only 2 lymph strips are applied from the left and right armpit to the cervico-thoracic junction (CTJ) area, where the strips cross over one another in the CTJ area. No new treatment appointments are then made, but it is agreed that the client will report as soon as she gets any symptoms.

After over a year the client makes contact again because of a similar symptom pattern. The treatment is then in accordance with the lymph treatment described. After three treatments she is again symptom free. For the last two years the client has remained symptom free.

5.3.3 Neck trauma, case 25

Case description:

A participant on the course tells how the evening before he was involved in a car accident. He was hit from the side. Initially there were no physical symptoms, but in the course of the following hours more and more pain and stiffness in the neck area developed.

During the first break on the course a rapid intervention with lymph tape was carried out, based on the assumption that microtrauma present caused the symptom build up. Depending on the reaction to this tape construction, in the course of the day it can always be decided to apply a more extensive, orthopaedic tape.

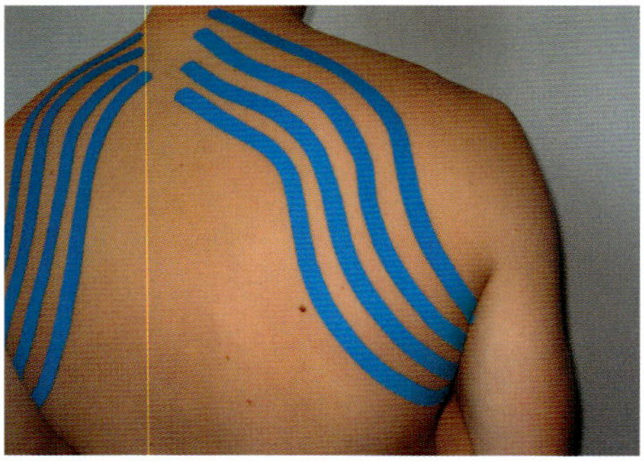

Bilateral lymph strips from the homolateral axillary to homolateral paravertebral.
Width of the tape strips: here ± 1.25 cm (5 cm wide tape cut into 4 strips).

The strips do not cross over one another in this case, because it was decided to tape peripheral from the problem area.

Because the reaction to a lymph tape builds up slowly, one also has to wait and see whether this tape construction gives the required result.
In the following hours the symptoms gradually diminish. It is therefore decided not to apply any further tapes at the moment.

5.3.4 Brachialgia, case 29

Case description:

During a course a course member states that he has had neck symptoms for some time already, where in particular the symptoms radiating to the right hand are bothersome. Due to physiotherapy the symptoms have diminished recently, but the tingling radiating to the fingers remains. Because the problem does not in fact fit in with the course being given at that time, a very short treatment is given during the break.

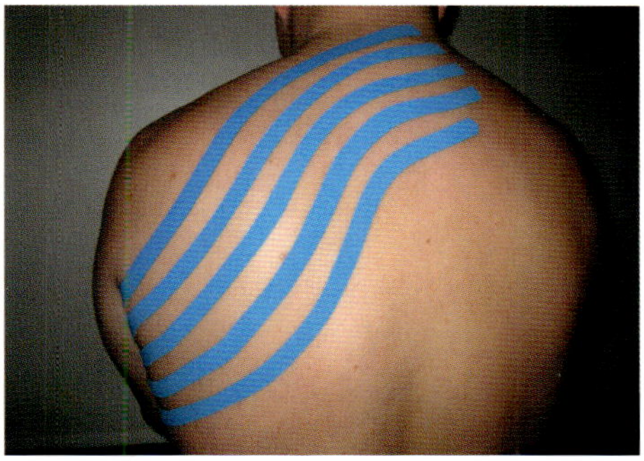

Lymph strips from the heterolateral axillary to the right side of the spine, low cervical and high thoracic.
Width of the tape strips: here ± 1.75 cm (5 cm wide tape cut into 4 strips).

Assuming that the homolateral drainage area may be overloaded by the constant irritation, it is decided here to make an anastomosis from the heterolateral armpit.

In the following hours the symptoms gradually diminish.
On the second day of the course, 14 days later, the symptoms appear to have considerably reduced. In the period with CureTape the symptoms have been entirely absent. However, after about ten days the tape started to work loose and had to be removed. After the removal of the tape the symptoms appeared to return but to a lesser extent.

On the second day of the course the course member was given an explanation of the tape method, so that he could continue the treatment at home for a while.

5.3.5 Back complaints lumbar spine, case 21

Case description:
A 65 year old woman comes into the practice because of back complaints. She has a long history of back complaints after a hernia 25 years ago. The hernia was treated surgically at the time, and afterwards treated in a rehabilitation centre. During this process it appears from the imaging material that two not fully closed low lumbar vertebral arches are involved.

Since the hernia operation she has never been entirely symptom free, the symptoms do vary in intensity. She suffers from morning stiffness, radiating symptoms to the lateral side of right leg and foot. She cannot lie on her right side at night because of the pain.

She has already been in treatment for some years by a physiotherapist/osteopath. This treatment usually helps a lot, but in the past 7 months seems to have brought no improvement. The osteopath thinks that the resistance to the treatment is partly caused by a fluid problem.

Since the hernia operation she has suffered from stress incontinence. She has been given medication for this for the last two years. She does in fact have the feeling that she is also retaining more fluid because of this medication.

Upon inspection an ample swelling in the lumbar area is visible, around the scar of the hernia operation.

Assuming that the local drainage area may be overloaded by the constant irritation, it is decided to make an anastomosis from the armpit. The strips from the left and right side cross over one another in the problem area, in this way the emphasis of the treatment is as far as possible located in the low lumbar area.

During the first treatment this lymph tape is combined with a tape to prevent stress incontinence and a ligament tape over the spine. Immediately after this tape lumbar flexion is easier to carry out and there is an increased range of motion.

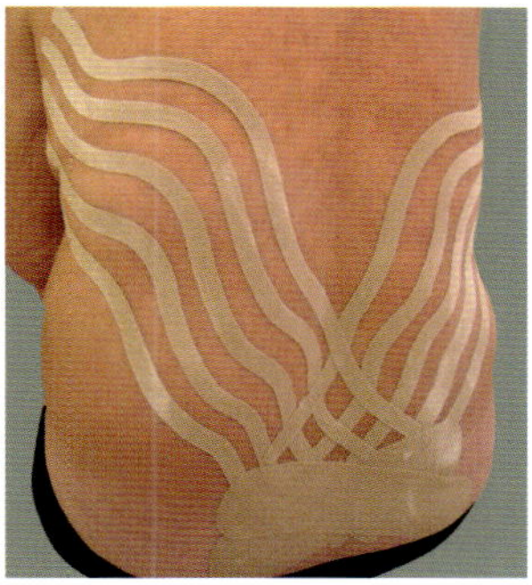

Bilateral lymph strips from both armpits, crossing in the problem area around the lumbar scar.
Width of the tape strips: here ± 1.25 cm (5 cm wide tape cut into 4 strips).

Upon evaluation of this treatment during the second appointment it appears that the ligament tape was however ultimately very poorly tolerated. The symptoms have otherwise diminished and she has been able to discontinue the medication for stress incontinence as long as the tape was present. Only the lymph tape and the tape to prevent the stress incontinence are therefore repeated.

During the following period the symptoms gradually diminish. After four treatments the frequency is reduced to one treatment every three weeks. The expectation is that this frequency can be reduced further and ultimately it will be enough to treat for a shorter time during more troublesome periods.

5.3.6 Abdominal complaints

In case of abdominal complaints where it is also assumed that the pressure of fluid in the abdominal cavity partly contributes to these symptoms or even causes the symptoms entirely, a well chosen lymph tape may bring relief. Also in case of IBS (irritable bowel syndrome) sometimes good results are achieved with lymph tape.

Normally the lymph from the abdominal area is drained below the navel via the inguinal lymph nodes and the lymph from the abdominal area above the navel via the axillary lymph nodes.

If there are symptoms due to pressure of fluid, there will usually be cause to assume that these normal drainage channels are overloaded. The choice to make an anastomosis with the lymph tapes is then obvious.

Depending on the situation more or less intensive treatment with tape will be chosen. In the treatment structure the first treatment will have a low intensity. Depending on the results the treatment after this may be intensified.

By taping to the lateral side of the abdomen, the drainage there is promoted which reduces the pressure. The lymph fluid will more readily move to a region with lower pressure.
The treatment can be intensified by using more strips that run further into the abdominal area.

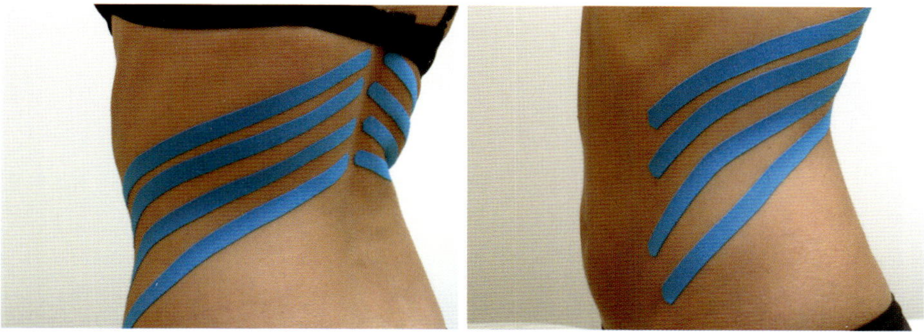

Bilateral anastomosis from homolateral paravertebral to the lateral side of the abdomen.
Width of the tape strips: here ± 1.25 cm (5 cm wide tape cut into 4 strips).

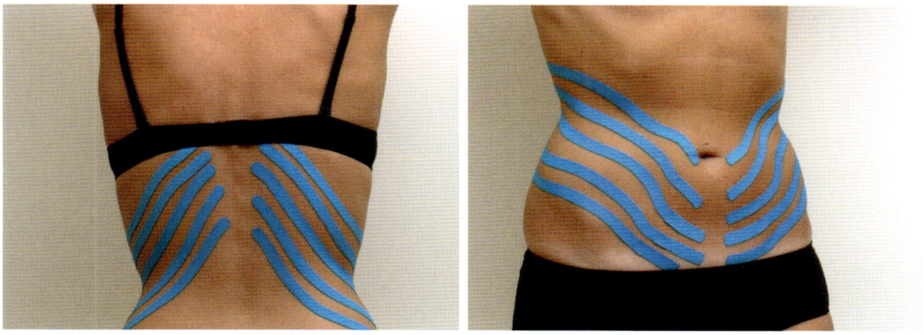

Bilateral anastomosis from homolateral paravertebral to the median line.
Width of the tape strips: here ± 1.25 cm (5 cm wide tape cut into 4 strips).

A further intensification can be achieved by having the strips cross with lymph strips from another drainage area, for example level with the sternum.

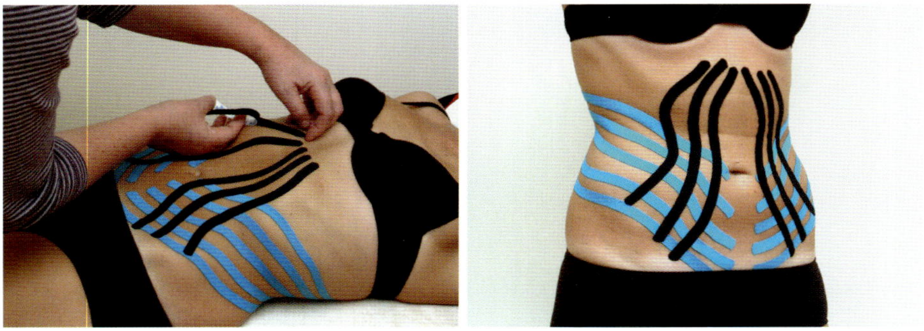

Bilateral anastomosis from homolateral paravertebral to the median line, combined with a bilateral anastomosis from the sternum into the lower abdomen.
Width of the tape strips: here ± 1.25 cm (5 cm wide tape cut into 4 strips).

More intensive treatment far from always gives the best treatment result. Sometimes intensive treatments are not well tolerated. It may also happen that due to more intensive treatment lymph actually moves into the problem area, which can even increase the symptoms.

N.B. Ascites may also be a symptom of the presence of benign or malignant tumours, liver conditions, kidney abnormalities, cardiac insufficiency, etc. Lymph taping is not advised if the cause of the abdominal complaints is insufficiently clear.

5.3.7 Gynaecological, post-operative, case 19

Case description:

A 54 year old woman has undergone a gynaecological operation. There is a post-operative haematoma and swelling present in the area of the operation. Under normal circumstances the abdominal area below the navel drains the lymph via the inguinal lymph nodes. Due to the operation wound this drainage path is obstructed after the operation.
Since CureTape is not sterile, the scar may only be taped over when the skin has fully closed. Before then it is of course possible to tape round the scar, for example by making an anastomosis with lymph strips from the armpit or from higher paravertebral to the cranial side of the scar.
From the underside lymph strips from the inguinal region to the caudal side of the scar can be used. Because of the location and the size of the scar the use of anastomosis tapes is made difficult here.
Once the scar has closed, tape can also be placed over the scar. This has the advantage that due to the lifting effect of the tape the growth of lymph vessels is promoted.

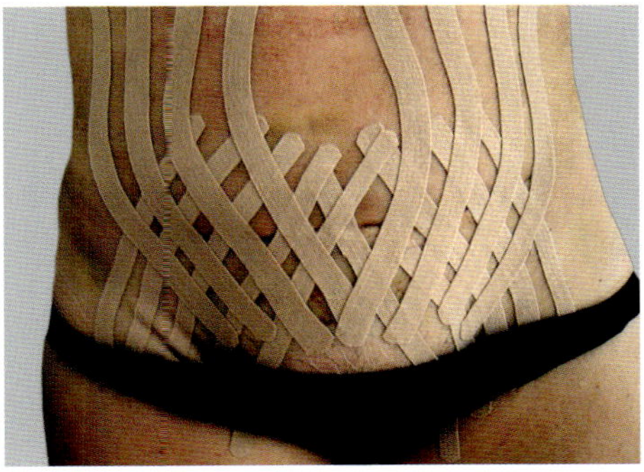

Bilateral anastomosis from the armpit to the os pubis, in the scar area crossing with lymph strips from the groin to just cranial from the scar.
Width of the tape strips: here ± 1.25 cm (5 cm wide tape cut into 4 strips).

Due to the tape treatment the haematoma is drained more quickly, the swelling is reduced more quickly and the scar heals better. Because the pressure in the operation area is reduced, at the same time the pain symptoms are diminished.
In this case three weeks after the operation no further tape treatment was necessary.

5.4 Upper extremity

5.4.1 Shoulder, Cuff rupture, case 6

Case description:

A 71 year old woman comes into the practice because of a cuff rupture in the left shoulder. Around ten months ago the GP twice injected corticosteroids because of a bursitis present. Two months after the last injection a spontaneous cuff rupture occurs during normal movement in ADL.

She has been in treatment for this problem with an orthopaedist and a physiotherapist. The orthopaedist considered the problem was inoperable and the physiotherapist has after a number of months said no further progress is anticipated. This client's question is whether Medical Taping could perhaps bring about a further improvement.

She has no pain when resting, but is sometimes woken up by the pain. In the examination it becomes clear that all active glenohumeral movements are greatly limited and painful. Careful muscle strength tests show a lot of problems in particular in abduction, anteflexion and exorotation direction.

The whole upper arm area is still swollen and still somewhat discoloured by the remains of the haematoma.

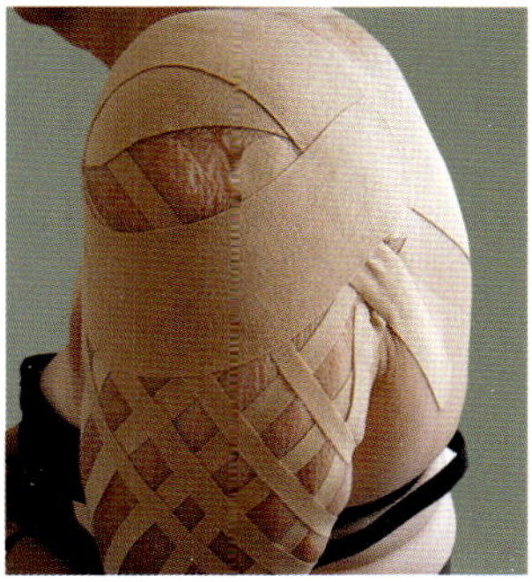

Lymph strips from heterolateral paravertebral via triceps/deltoid area to biceps, and lymph strips from homolateral supraclavicular via biceps/deltoid to the triceps. Here a combination with orthopaedic tapes, the lymph strips are always applied first.
Width of the tape strips: here ± 1 cm (5 cm wide tape cut into 5 strips).

The client remains in treatment for a long time. Due to the tape treatment the swelling disappears and the movement possibilities during ADL do increase, but a considerable residual symptom remains present. Ultimately the situation becomes acceptable and stable, as long as the stabilising glenohumeral tape is used.

The husband learns to apply this tape and after four months the wife leaves treatment. The husband continues applying the taping at home.

Orthopaedic tapes used here: posture correction, detoning M. Teres minor, stabilising glenohumeral.

Note: a so-called 'more mature skin' may have wrinkles. These wrinkles must be smoothed with the hand during taping to prevent skin irritation.

5.4.2 Shoulder complaints, case 14

Case description:

The 40 year old client has already been under treatment for some time with breaks because of hyper mobility syndrome. This time she comes into the practice after a recent trauma in which she has fallen and received shoulder symptoms.

Ventral from the glenohumeral joint a swelling is present, but further investigation is hampered by the pain symptoms present. Because the swelling present very probably substantially contributes to the pain symptoms and also prevents investigation, first of all treatment is started to reduce the swelling.

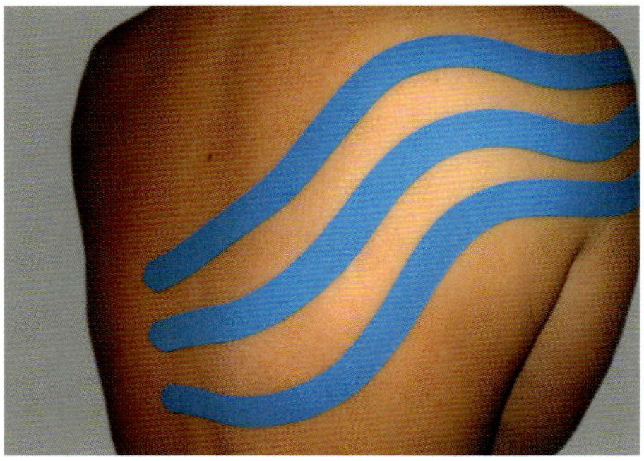

Anastomosis from paravertebral heterolateral to the front of the glenohumeral joint.
Width of the tape strips: here ± 1.65 cm (5 cm wide tape cut into 3 strips).

The lymph drainage from the ventral shoulder area under normal circumstances runs via the axillary lymph nodes and to a lesser degree via the supraclavicular lymph nodes. Since this area seems overloaded, it was decided here to use anastomosis from heterolateral paravertebral.

Somewhat wider tape strips are used, because the slightly wider tape can often be left in position for a little longer.

After the swelling had reduced, the examination could be carried out and adequate treatment started.

5.4.3 Lower arm fracture

In the case of a fracture it may be sensible to apply lymph tape proximal from the plaster. The swelling present is hereby controlled and a contribution made to preventing the plaster getting too tight, which can put the blood supply at risk.

Depending on the situation a more or less intensive tape construction may be decided on.

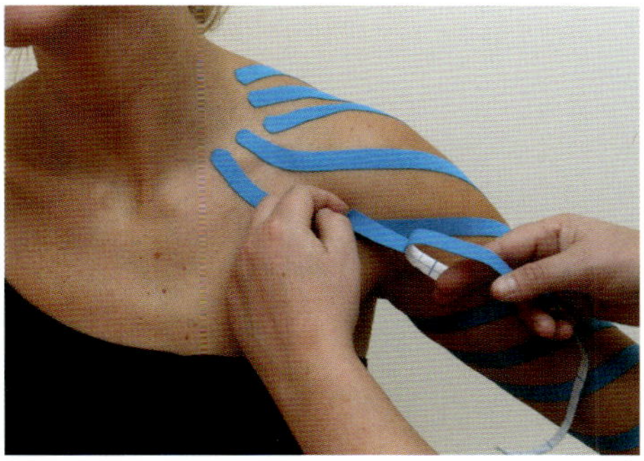

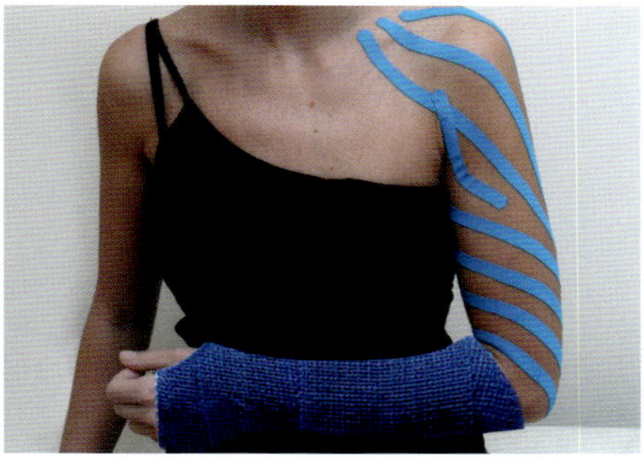

Lymph strips from homolateral supraclavicular to just under the upper edge of the plaster.
Width of the tape strips: here ± 1.25 cm (5 cm wide tape cut into 4 strips).

The treatment may be made more intensive by building up an extra lymph tape, in which all the strips cross the previous strips.

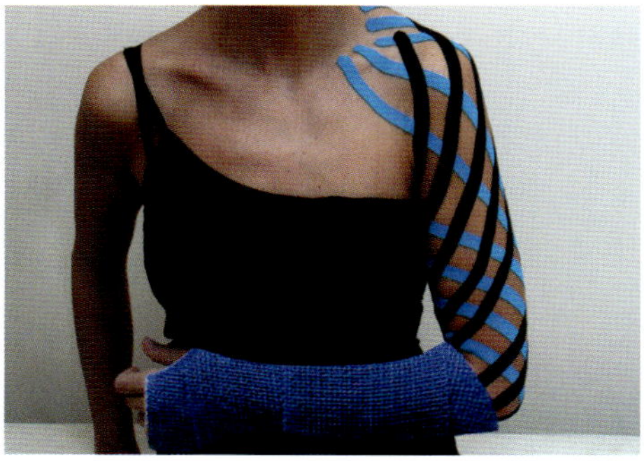 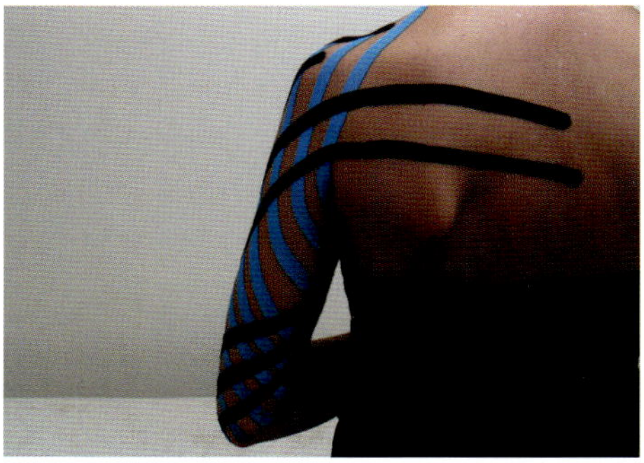

Lymph strips from homolateral supraclavicular to just under the upper edge of the plaster, then cross-wise lymph strips that are partly positioned from homolateral supraclavicular and partly as anastomosis from homolateral paravertebral.
Width of the tape strips: here ± 1.25 cm (5 cm wide tape cut into 4 strips).

Although in this example taping is mainly carried out from the homolateral supraclavicular area, the use of anastomoses in such situations is often sensible. Once it is suspected that lymph drainage along the usual pathway may be hampered because this area is overloaded, anastomosis must be decided on. If anastomosis is used, the tape strips may for example be positioned from the heterolateral armpit or from paravertebral.

N.B. The photo model did not have a broken arm at the time of the photo session, the photos were touched up later when the arm plaster was added.

5.4.4 Wrist fracture, case 17

Case description:
A 53 year old hairdresser fell when skating. At the First Aid post a crack was found in the processus styloideus of the left radius. A plaster splint was made to measure, because the considerable swelling and haematoma present made a full plaster impossible.
During the first treatment taping was carried out proximal from the plaster splint with lymph strips from homolateral supraclavicular. Four days after this tape treatment the swelling was sufficiently reduced to fit a full plaster. After four weeks in plaster this can be removed and she comes into the practice for further treatment.
At that time there is still moderate local swelling. The movement possibilities in the wrist joint are limited in all directions. Furthermore the pinching strength has clearly been reduced, the extension of the fingers is slightly restricted and the thumb movements are restricted in adduction and extension direction.
With narrow lymph strips a local grid is constructed over the swelling. After this muscle tapes are used to tone both the extensor group and the flexor group and a ligament tape to support the wrist as far as possible.

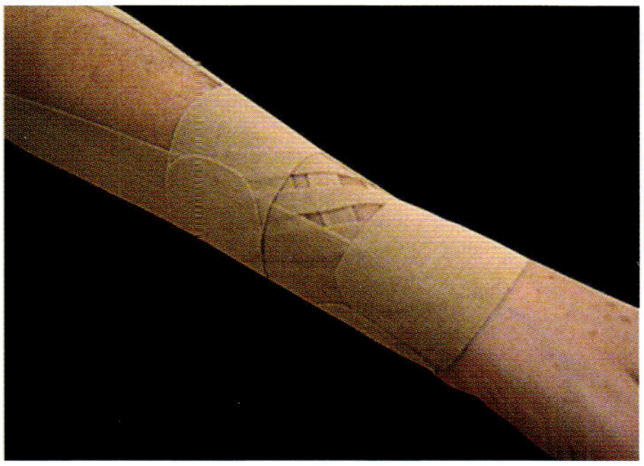

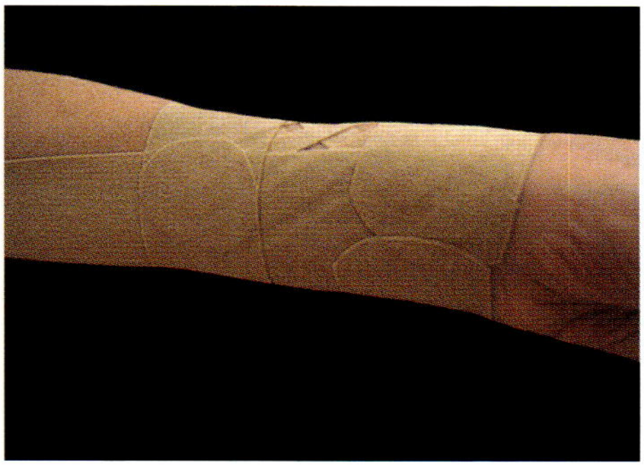

Local crossing lymph strips from proximal to peripheral, combined with orthopaedic tapes. Width of the lymph strips: here ±1 cm (5 cm wide tape cut into 5 strips).

Note: the tape strip proximal from the grid is only applied to reinforce the end of the grid tapes. On the distal side the ligament tape has this function.

5.4.5 Bursitis olecrani

There are various possibilities for treating a local swelling with lymph taping, such as for example in case of a bursitis olecrani. These methods differ mainly in intensity of the treatment (see § 4.8.1).

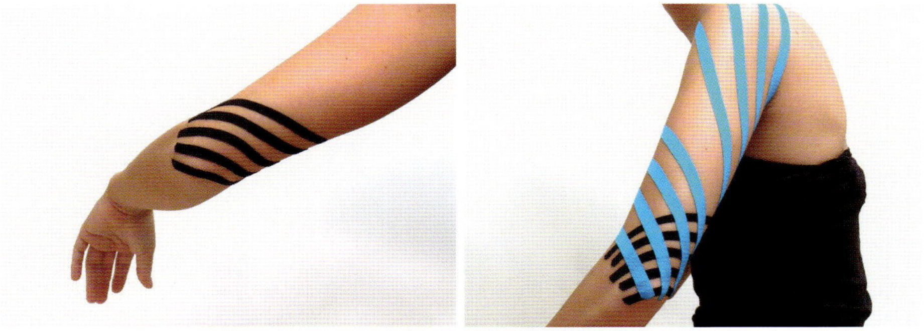

Photo left: local lymph strips, applied parallel from proximal to distal
Photo right: local parallel lymph strips, combined with longer lymph strips from homolateral supraclavicular which cross the local strips, so that the emphasis of the treatment is local.
Width of the lymph strips: the local strips ±1 cm wide, the longer strips ± 1.25 cm wide (5 cm wide tape cut into respectively 5 and 4 strips).

Bursitis olecrani, case 18

A client, 38 years, with a swelling in the bursa of the right olecranon as a result of a trauma. During the trauma shoulder injury has occurred on the same side. This shoulder injury seems to be more severe than the swelling around the elbow and is therefore given priority within the treatment. There is moderate swelling around the olecranon. Both reasons play a part in the decision to work locally.

In this case two crossing fan-shaped tapes are decided on. A fan-shaped tape is taken here, because the wider base of the fan comes loose slightly less easily than the narrow base of separate and separately positioned parallel strips.

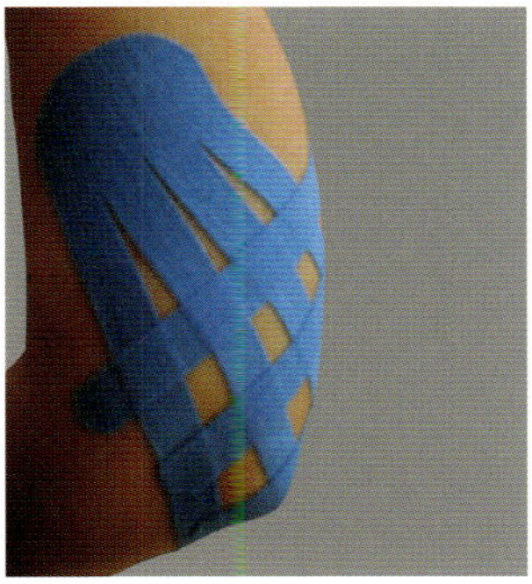

Locally applied, crossing fan-shaped tapes, from proximal to distal.
Width of the tape strips: here ± 1.25 cm (5 cm wide tape cut into 4 strips).

After two treatments the swelling around the olecranon has disappeared. The shoulder injury required two more extra treatments.

5.4.6 Tennis elbow, case 8

Case description:

This involves the same client as described in § 5.3.1. For a more detailed description of this case please refer to the relevant paragraph.

In first instance this seems to concern a 'pure' epicondylitis lateralis, treatment is therefore initially only around the elbow.

Because there is swelling present around the elbow, the classic orthopaedic epicondylitis lateralis tape is combined with lymph tape. The lymph strips are in such a case always applied first, the orthopaedic tapes are then applied over them.

In the first treatment it was decided to use locally applied lymph tape. Because at the second treatment it appears that the swelling was insufficiently reduced, the lymph tape is then applied more intensively.

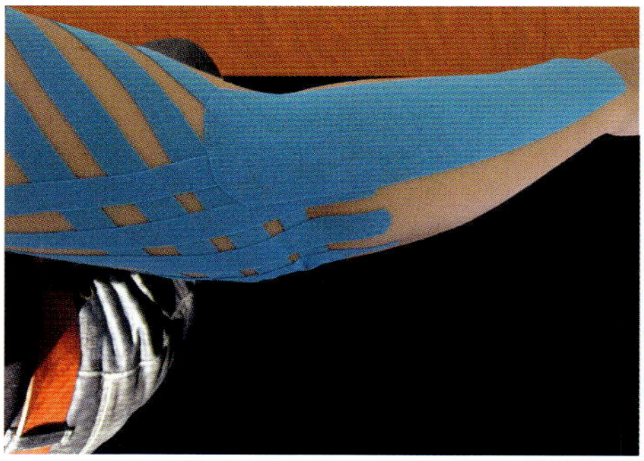

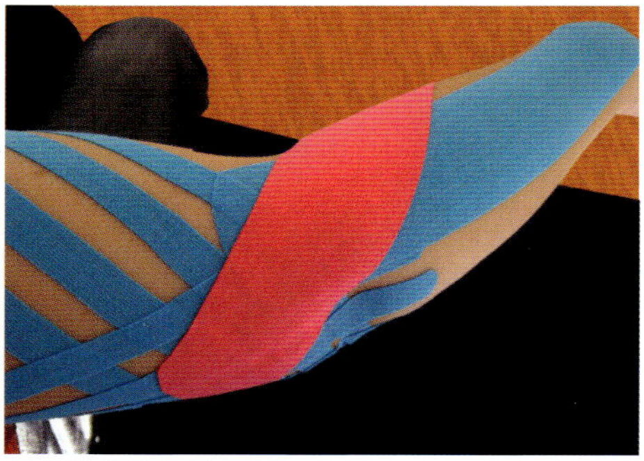

Lymph strips from supraclavicular, where 4 strips from ventral and four strips from dorsal cross one another locally and form a local grid. The emphasis of the treatment lies on the local swelling. Here combined with a classic epicondylitis lateralis tape.

Width of the lymph strips: here around 1.25 cm (5 cm wide tape cut into 4 strips).

Ultimately the treatment only appears to give a good and lasting result after a combination is made with a cervical treatment. After a total of five treatments the client is symptom free.

5.4.7 Dystrophy lower arm

In particular in the first stage of reflex dystrophy good to very good results are seen when intensive lymph taping is used. In the second and third stage of this process the treatment results of lymph taping are much less good.

The biggest problem in the treatment of dystrophy in the first stage may be that there is possibly severe hyperaesthesia, as a result of which the tape cannot be tolerated. Unfortunately there is still no solution for this problem.

If the tape can be tolerated however, an intensive, crossed lymph tape is applied over the local area. The treatment can still be intensified a little more by working with longer strips from more proximal.
The tape is constructed from proximal to distal, the strips run to the wrist crease, even if it is wanted to treat the hand as well. The hand in fact forms an exception, see below.

Tape structure:

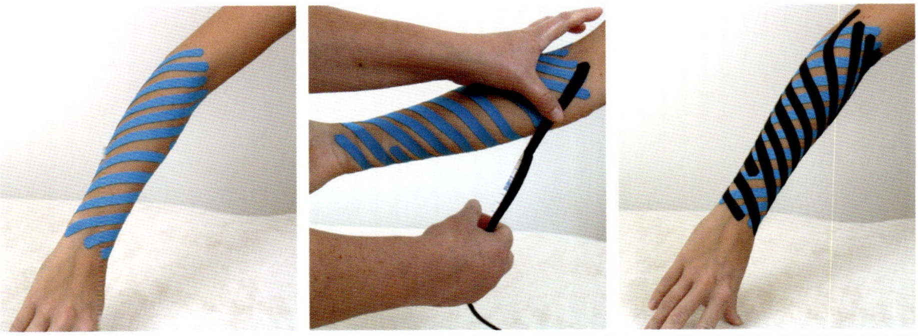

Photo left: lymph strips applied parallel from the elbow socket to the wrist fold. Photo middle: crossing lymph strips applied parallel from the elbow socket to the wrist fold. Photo right: completed tape.
Width of the lymph strips: here ± 1.25 cm (5 cm wide tape cut into 4 strips).

In practice it has been found that this tape construction is sufficient for the treatment. Experience to date is that if in fact treatment can be carried out in this way, the dystrophy process is effectively counteracted and within three to five treatments is no longer present.

If it is wanted to treat the hand as well, it must be taken into account that empirically it has been found that the hand _usually_ forms an exception when lymph taping and taping must be carried out from distal to proximal. See also the following paragraph.

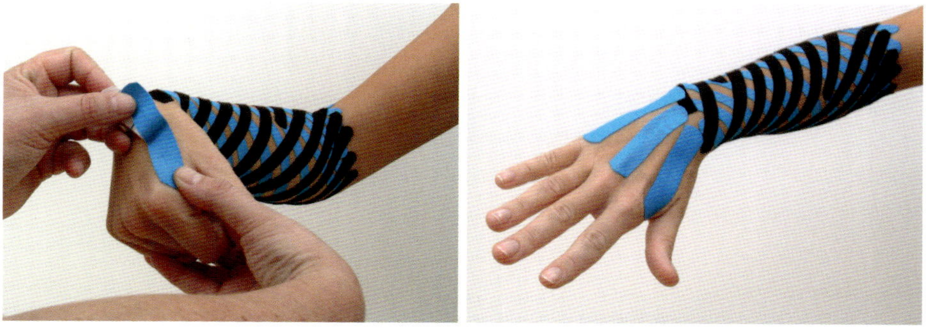

Lymph tape lower arm combined with a lymph tape of the hand. The lymph strips are applied to the hand from the base of the fingers to the wrist fold.
Width of the lymph strips on the hand: here ± 1.65 cm (5 cm wide tape cut into 3 strips).

In case of dystrophy in the lower extremity a similar treatment can be given (see also § 5.5.7).

5.4.8 Hand

If a swelling of the hand and/or the fingers must be treated, one should take into account that empirically it has been found that the hand usually forms an exception in lymph taping. In the great majority of cases lymph tape from distal to proximal on the back of the hand gives the best treatment result.

The reason for this is not entirely clear. It is assumed that the lymph in the network of lymph vessels in the hand flows more readily round the metacarpalia to the palm side and from there can be drained to the lower arm.

A logical conclusion could therefore be to tape the hand on the palm side. The practical problem is however that a palm tape will work loose much more quickly than a dorsal hand tape.

To make things even more difficult, this exception does not always apply. In some cases the hand must also be taped from proximal to distal. This cannot be determined in advance. The most pragmatic thing is therefore to warn the client at the first treatment that the tape should be removed from the hand immediately if the swelling in the hand seems to be increasing. At the following treatment taping can then be carried out in the other direction.

Examples of lymph tapes on the hand:

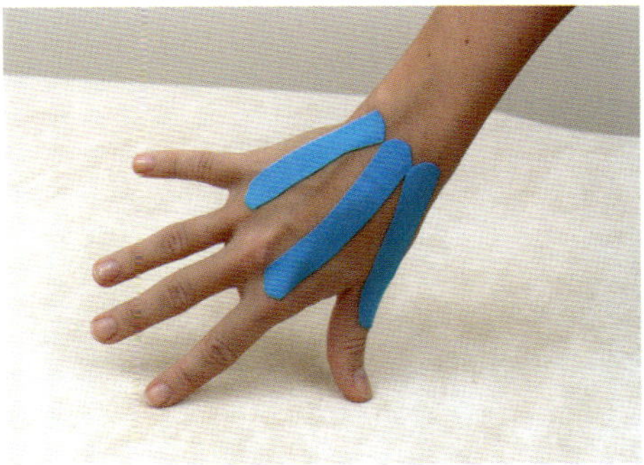

Parallel lymph strips on the hand, applied from the base of the fingers to the wrist crease.
Width of the lymph strips: here ± 1.65 cm (5 cm wide tape cut into 3 strips).

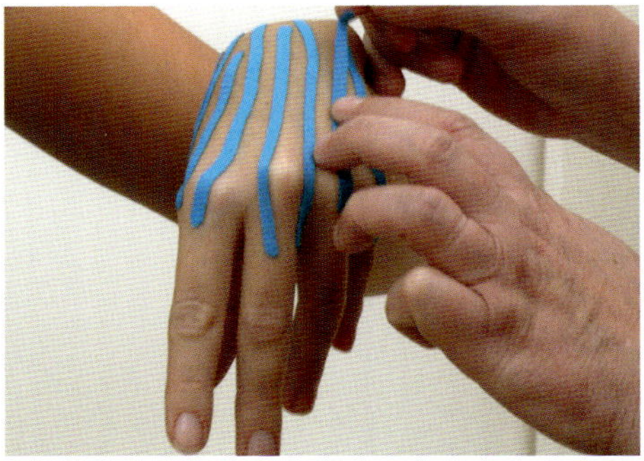

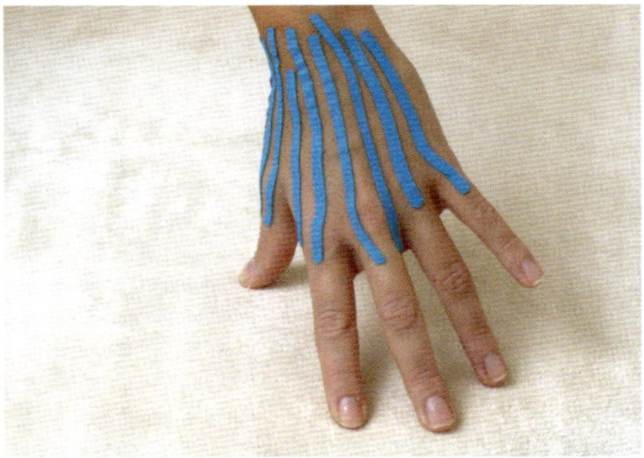

Parallel lymph strips on the hand, applied from the base of the fingers to the wrist crease.
Width of the lymph strips: here ± 0.6 cm (5 cm wide tape cut into 8 strips).

The narrower strips are in fact more effective, but work loose more easily. Because a tape on the back of the hand in any case already works loose more quickly, this may be a reason to work with somewhat wider strips on the back of the hand.

116

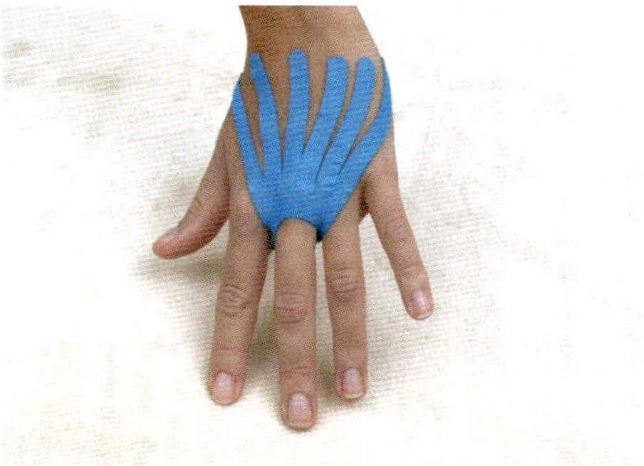

Fan-shaped lymph tape from the middle finger. A hole is cut in the base of the tape, so that this can be pushed around the middle finger.
Width of the lymph strips: here ± 0.8 cm (5 cm wide tape cut into 6 strips).

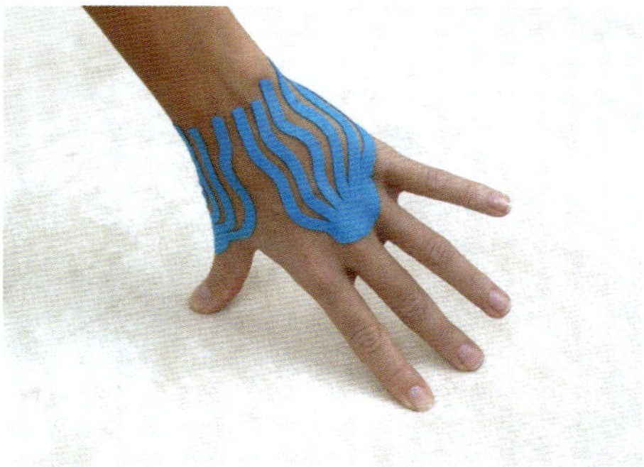

Fan-shaped lymph tape, applied in wavelike form, from the base of the middle finger. For the thumb a similar tape to treat the entire back of the hand.
Width of the lymph strips: here ± 0.8 cm (5 cm wide tape cut into 6 strips), for the thumb also ± 0.8 cm (2.5 cm wide tape cut into 3 strips).

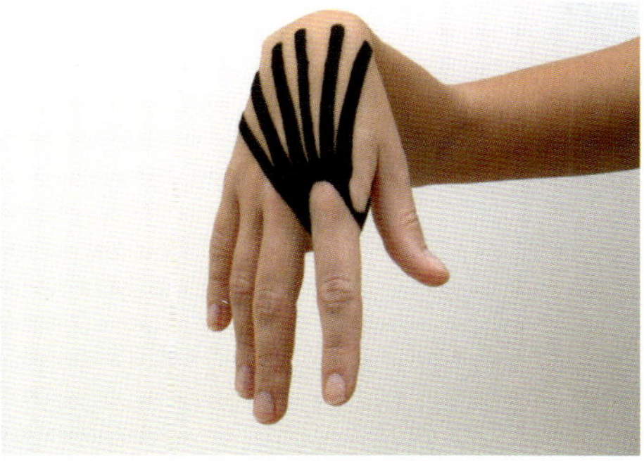

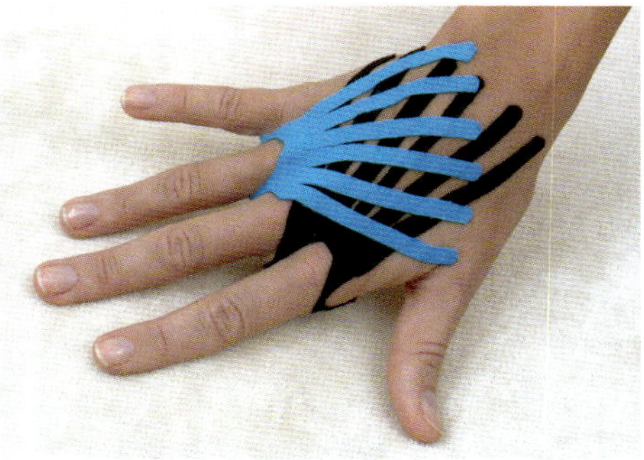

Crossed fan-shaped lymph tape from the index finger and the ring finger. In the base of the tape a hole is cut, so that this can be pushed around the finger.
Width of the lymph strips: here ± 0.8 cm (5 cm wide tape cut into 6 strips).

The choice for a lymph tape on the hand will mainly be based on practical considerations. Fan-shaped tapes are more difficult to apply, particularly those whose base is positioned around the finger. Parallel strips are if necessary easier to replace by the client themselves. Because a tape always works loose more quickly on the back of the hand, this latter consideration may be important.

5.4.9 Fingers, case 10

Case description:
A 49 year old man comes into the practice after an operation. In a trauma he has suffered a so-called 'ski-thumb' on the right, which ultimately, after over 10 months, was operated on. After the operation he is treated further with a plaster splint.

Around 5 months after the original trauma the second and third fingers in particular suddenly swelled up. A blood test and an examination by the neurologist gave no clue as to the cause of this swelling.

The operation has had no effect on the swelling of the fingers, in either a positive or negative sense. His question is whether something can be done about the finger swelling using Medical Taping.

By comparison the fourth and the fifth fingers also appear to be swollen, but to a lesser extent than the second and third fingers. The lymph tape is applied locally, distal from the plaster splint.

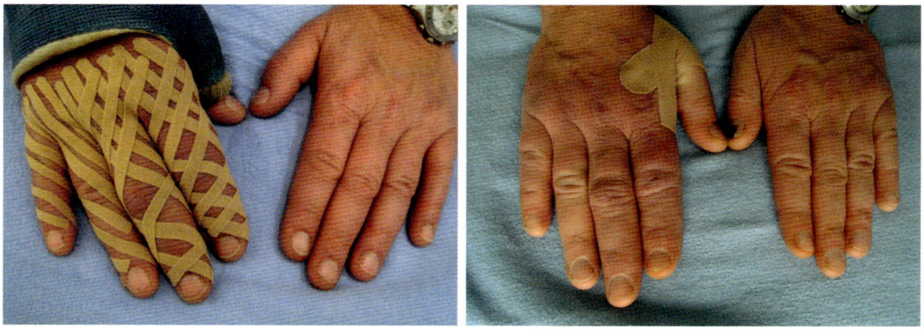

Parallel lymph strips over the fingers, applied from proximal to distal. Because the second and third fingers are clearly more severely swollen, a more intensive lymph tape is used there, namely crossed parallel tapes. Photo right: treatment result after four weeks.

Width of the lymph strips: here ± 0.6 cm (5 cm wide tape cut into 8 strips).

Although the lymph tapes on the fingers have reduced in size, after four weeks the treatment result is still not enough. The possibility is considered that in the original trauma local lymph collectors were also damaged.

Upon a further blood test however an infection with Lyme's disease is found to be present. Suitable treatment for this is started, after which the swelling in the fingers disappears.

5.4.10 Mallet Finger, case 30

Case description:

During a course a participant is present with a finger splint. The dorsal aponeurosis has torn spontaneously, for which she has been given this splint. She will in any case have to wear the splint for 6 weeks, of which there are still five weeks to go. Because the splint is very much in the way for her daily activities, her question is whether treatment with Medical Taping could replace the splint.

The swelling present is first treated with lymph tape, over this comes the orthopaedic tape for correction and support.

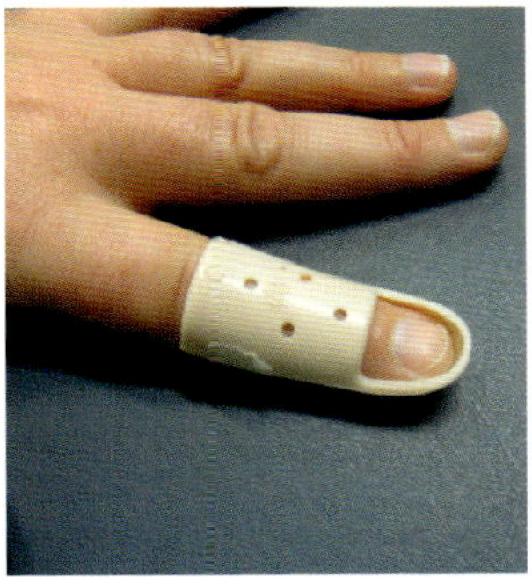
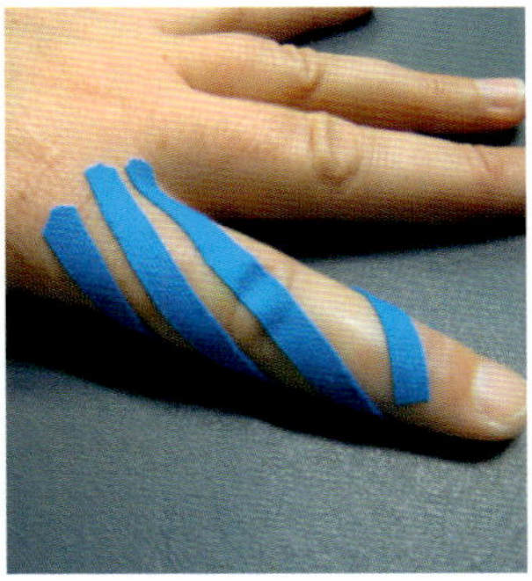
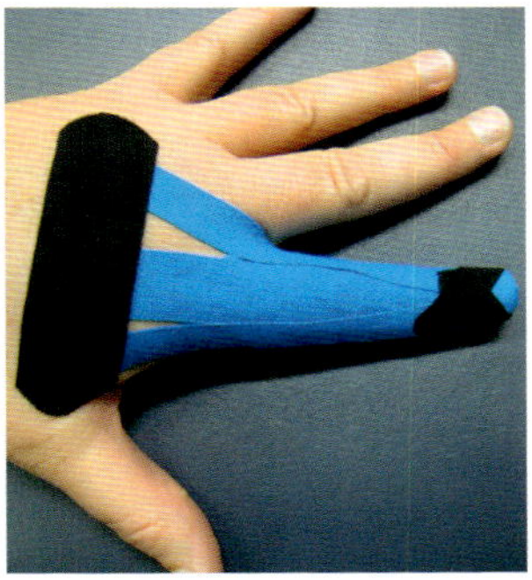

Photo left: splint for Mallet finger.
Photo middle: parallel lymph strips index finger from proximal to peripheral.
Photo right: combined with orthopaedic tapes for support.
Width of the lymph strips: here ± 0.6 cm (5 cm wide tape cut into 8 strips).

During the second day of the course, two weeks later, it appears that she has gone back to wearing the splint. Because with Medical Taping the possibility of movement is maintained, the tape treatment did not feel safe enough for her.

The finger swelling has reduced. She is also planning to use the Medical Taping method for support during the period when the splint can be removed.

5.5 Lower extremity

5.5.1 Hip, case 23

Case description:

A participant on a two day course has around two weeks beforehand had an accident, in which he has fallen on his right side. Gradually after the accident a considerable swelling has developed by the trochanter and distal from the trochanter. There is no visible haematoma and to date there is little response to manual lymph drainage.

On the first day of the course he asks whether treatment with Medical Taping could contribute to recovery.

In view of the size of the swelling and the fact that to date the effect of manual lymph drainage has been moderate, it is decided to use anastomoses.

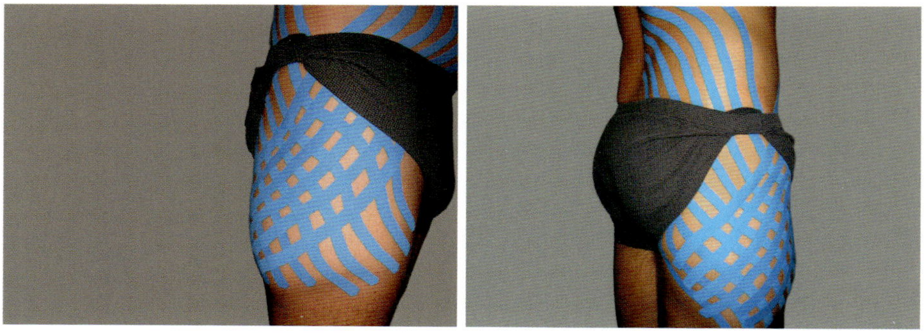

Lymph strips from the sternum and from paravertebral, crossing in the problem area. Width of the lymph strips: here ± 1.25 cm (5 cm wide tape cut into 4 strips).

At the start of the second day, around 15 hours after the treatment with lymph taping, he says that it already feels 'easier' and 'lighter'. At the end of the second day of the course, around 24 hours after the treatment, he is enthusiastic about the result and determined to continue the treatment at home. It is not known whether this in fact happened and what the result ultimately was.

5.5.2 Hydrops knee

A hydrops in the knee can be treated effectively in various ways with a lymph tape construction. The methods differ mainly in intensity (see also § 4.8.1). Several considerations can play a part in the choice of the method used.

Under more taxing circumstances, for example due to use of medication or underlying pathology, the choice will tend to be for a more intensive lymph tape. In case of hydrops a combination with orthopaedic tapes will often be wanted, and that may also play a part in the ultimate choice of treatment.

During taping the knee is preferably brought to maximum flexion, to create stretch in the skin. The round shape hampers the application of an even lymph tape.

<u>Hydrops art. genu, example 1</u>
Local treatment of hydrops.

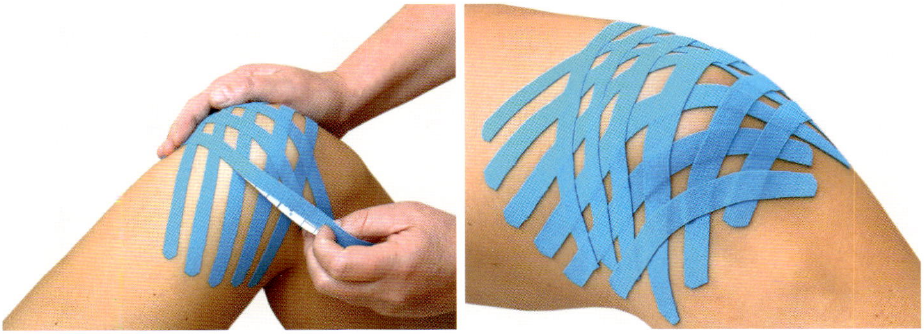

Crossing local lymph strips, applied from proximal to distal.
Width of the lymph strips: here ± 1.25 cm (5 cm wide tape cut into 4 strips).

Hydrops art. genu, example 2

The treatment can be extended by having lymph strips from a more proximal located drainage area end just in the local crossed lymph tape. Taping can for example be carried out from the inguinal area.

If it is expected that the inguinal area will not be adequately able to process the quantity of lymph produced, or in the case of hip and/or abdominal complaints, these may be reasons to work with anastomoses. The lymph strips can then for example be applied from paravertebral.

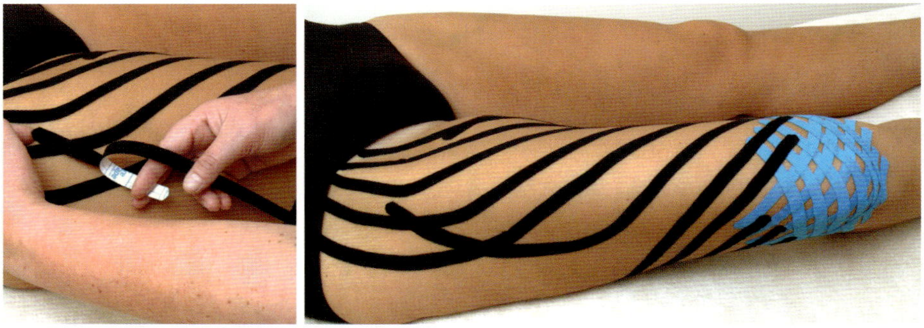

Lymph strips from the inguinal area, ending just in the local crossed lymph tape.
Width of the lymph strips: here ± 1.25 cm (5 cm wide tape cut into 4 strips).

If it is not possible to stretch the skin sufficiently due to movement restrictions present or due to the uncomfortable starting position, this cannot be offset by using more stretch in the lymph strips. In that case the skin must be stretched more with the fingers in a proximal direction.

In the treatment described the emphasis of the lymph tape lies on the ventral side of the knee. The lymph strips can also be positioned in the popliteal area, taping is then carried out with the knee in extension.

Another method of reducing the tension in the popliteal area is by using an X-tape on the dorsal side of the knee. This X-tape is applied in extension, which stretches the skin.
The tape itself is applied without additional stretch, but maintaining pretensioning.

The paper is torn in the middle, after which the tape is applied in the popliteal area. The four ends are positioned slightly to the outside.

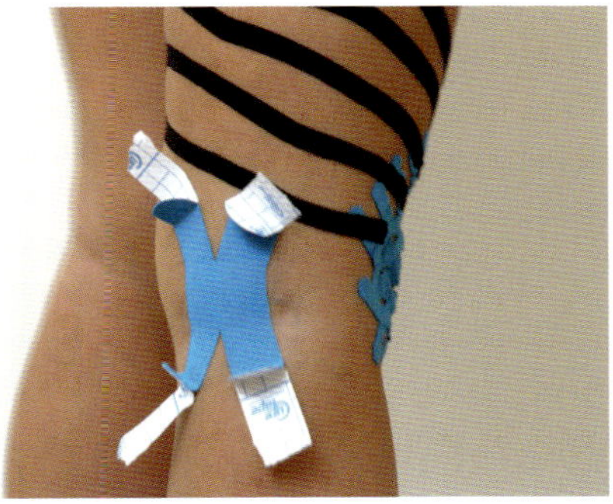

X-tape to reduce pressure in the popliteal area.
Width of the tape: 5 cm wide tape cut into an X shape. Length: ± 12 to 15 cm.

Hydrops art. genu, example 3

Another method for constructing a similar treatment is by applying local parallel lymph strips, which are crossed by lymph strips from a proximal located drainage area.

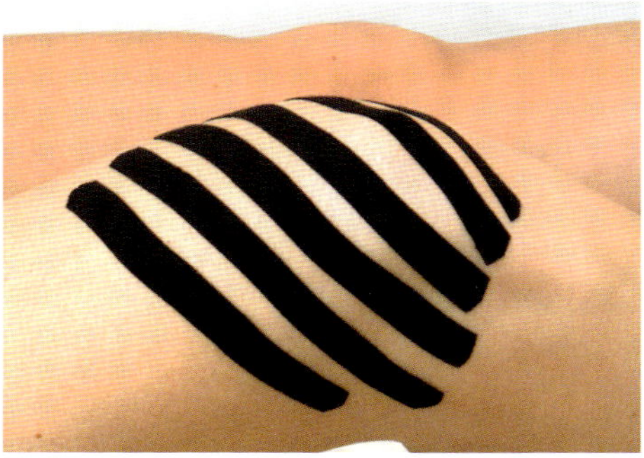

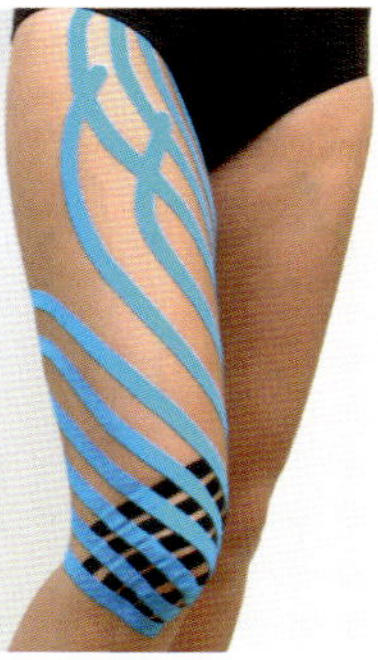

Local parallel lymph strips, applied from proximal to distal, which are crossed by longer lymph strips from inguinal.

Width of the lymph strips: here ± 1.25 cm (5 cm wide tape cut into 4 strips).

Here too the emphasis lies on treatment on the ventral side of the knee and the lymph tape can be extended with an X-tape on the dorsal side as described.

The choice for the tape construction from example 2 or the tape construction from example 3 is primarily an individual one. Both tape constructions will show a corresponding action.

5.5.3 Cruciate ligament plasty, case 27

Case description:

A participant in a two day course had five days previously undergone a front cruciate ligament plasty on the right knee. Although the recovery is going well and she has noticeably few symptoms, there is still a relatively moderate swelling present and the remains of the haematoma are visible. Her question is whether Medical Taping could support the recovery further.

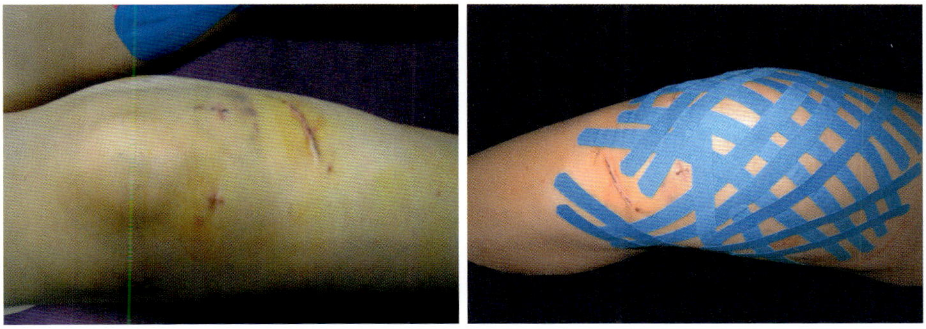

Photo left: initial situation: the operation scars have not yet healed, the adhesions are still present. Photo right: local crossing lymph strips from the upper leg to the haematoma by the tibial plateau.

Width of the lymph strips: here ± 1.25 cm (5 cm wide tape cut into 4 strips).

In view of the good recovery and the relatively moderate swelling, it is decided to use local taping, although with slightly longer lymph strips. Because the operation scars have not yet fully healed, they cannot yet be taped over. The lymph strips are applied such that the whole area is reached, while the scars remain free of tape.

This tape construction is felt by her to give virtually immediate relief. Subjectively there is also a virtually immediate increase in the range of movement in a flexion direction.

5.5.4 Arthrolith, case 28

Case description:

A 52 year old logistics manager comes into the practice because of right knee complaints. The symptoms have recently arisen, without any clear previous trauma. This involves pain that occurs suddenly from time to time and for a short duration. When there are pain symptoms, the knee is 'locked' and further movement is temporarily not possible. The knee has not been red or hot, there is some swelling present however.

The examination gives little specific evidence, since at that time no symptoms are present. The range of movement is slightly restricted in a flexion direction and a moderate hydrops is palpable.

The working hypothesis is to assume the presence of an arthrolith. The treatment is a combination of a local lymph tape with orthopaedic tapes for support.

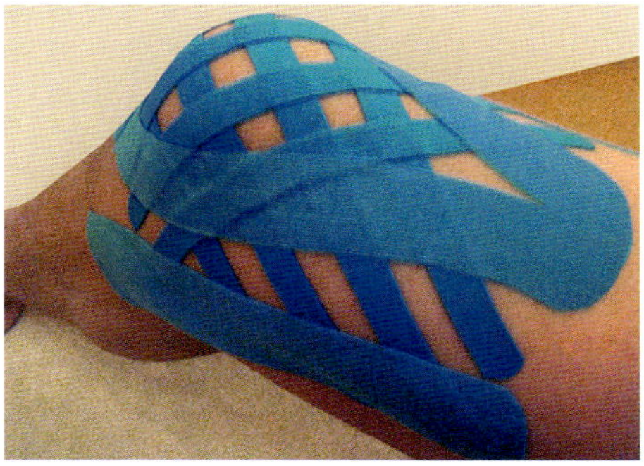

Local crossing lymph tapes, applied from proximal to distal. Combination with ligament support of the joint and a proprioceptive patella tape.
Width of the lymph strips: here ± 1.25 cm (5 cm wide tape cut into 4 strips).

He cancelled the second treatment, because the symptoms had not returned and the swelling is no longer present. Upon telephone follow-up after three weeks it appears that the symptoms have not reoccurred.

5.5.5 Ankle distortion

A lymph tape to counteract a swelling after an ankle distortion can be composed in a similar way to the lymph tape construction described in § 5.4.5 (bursitis olecrani) and § 5.5.2 (hydrops art. genu).
Here a local crossed lymph tape is shown on the lateral side of the ankle. Of course the whole swelling must be taped, also on the medial side if swelling is present there.
In case of an acute ankle injury taping is carried out in the pain free state. If as a result it is not possible to stretch the skin sufficiently, the skin must be stretched with the hand in a proximal direction (see § 4.6.1).

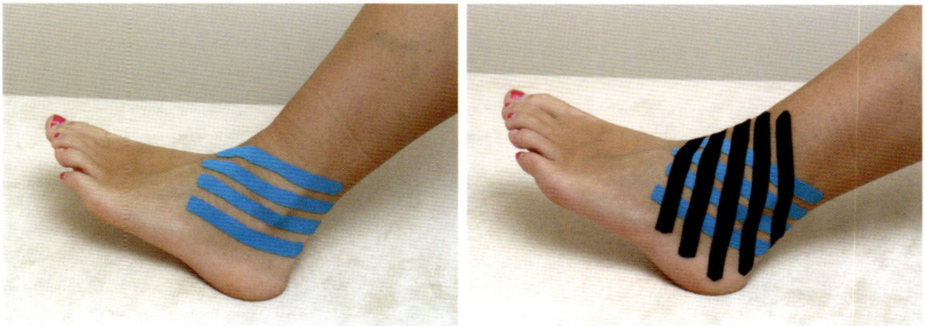

Crossed local lymph tapes, applied from proximal to distal.
Width of the lymph strips: here ± 1.25 cm (5 cm wide tape cut into 4 strips).

The action of the lymph tape can be made more intensive by having longer lymph strips from proximal end in the local lymph tape.

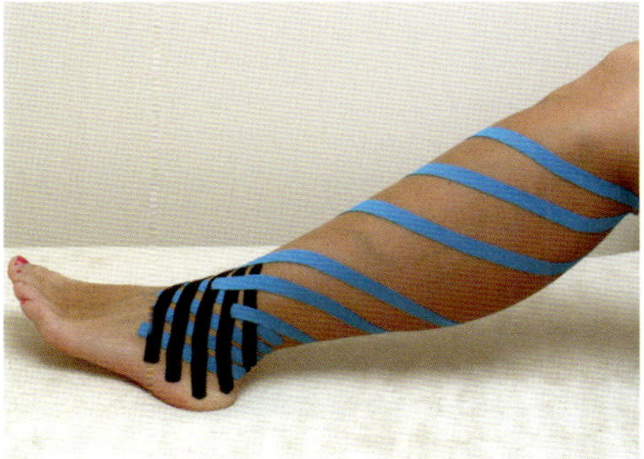

Parallel lymph strips from the knee, just ending in the local lymph tape.
Width of the lymph strips: here ± 1.25 cm (5 cm wide tape cut into 4 strips).

5.5.6 Inversion trauma, case 16

Case description:

During a course a participant asks whether there is room for treatment. One of her family members had had an inversion trauma two days before, at the moment he is walking with two crutches. On the X-ray photo no fracture was visible. This man is then treated during the course.

There is considerable swelling on the medial and lateral side. The foot can as a result not be brought sufficiently to dorsal flexion. Because of the swelling present a further examination is not possible at the moment, the emphasis of the treatment lies on bringing down the swelling.

The choice is for a lymph tape, constructed from the popliteal region. The lymph strips from the lateral side of the knee are positioned in a spiral to the medial side of the ankle, the lymph strips from the medial side of the knee are positioned in a spiral to the lateral side of the ankle. In this way the whole ankle joint is treated with lymph tapes.

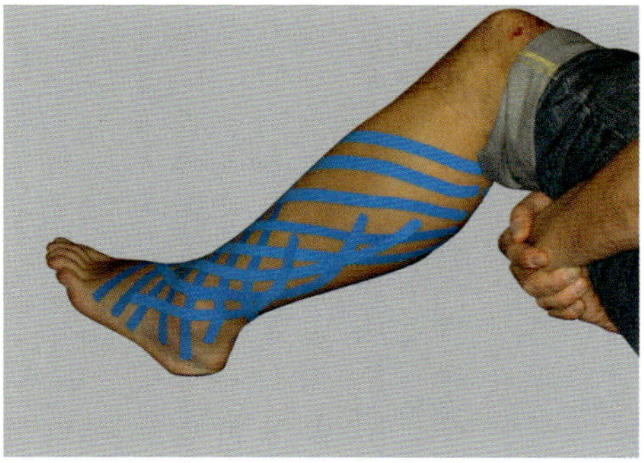

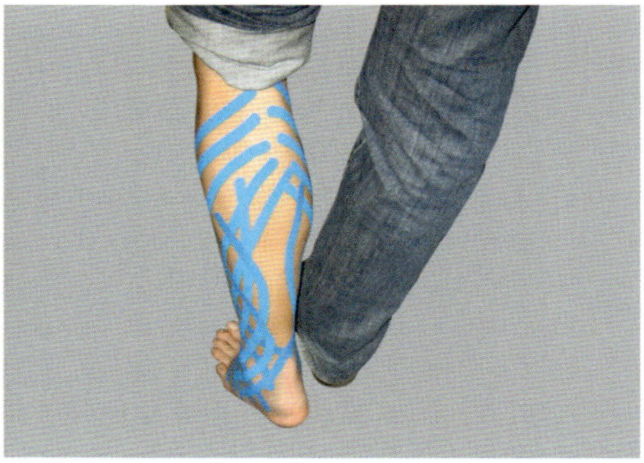

Lymph strips from the popliteal region, crossing on the ventral side of the leg and around the ankle.

Width of the lymph strips: here ± 1.25 cm (5 cm wide tape cut into 4 strips).

The lymph strips do not all start exactly from the popliteal area, but are applied spread out from the popliteal area and proximal in the calf. This avoided a concentration of tape in the popliteal area.

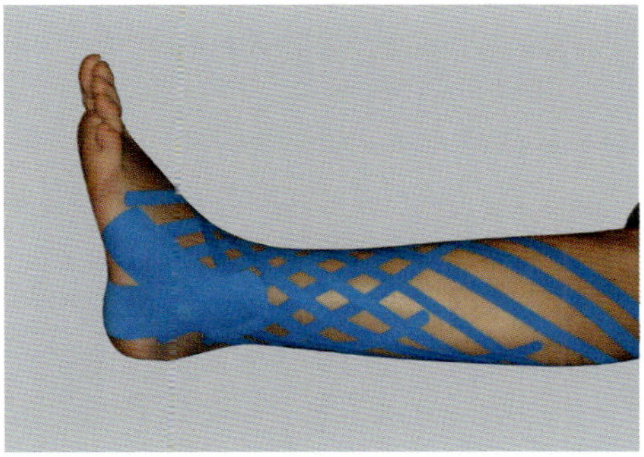

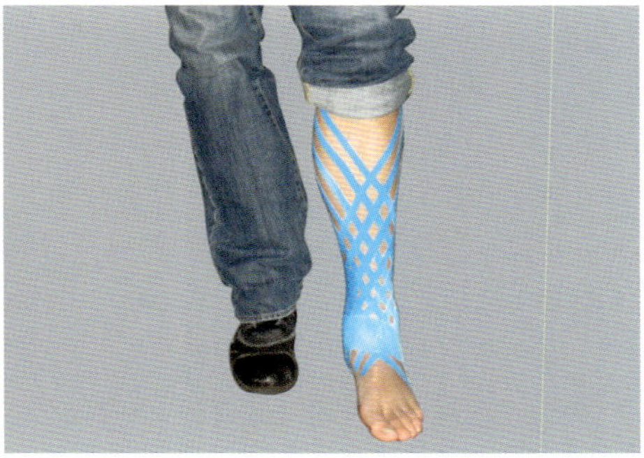

Combination with adapted orthopaedic tapes to stabilise the ankle.
Photo right: shows that the tape has talcum powder rubbed into it. This is to prevent it coming lose prematurely.

Around a quarter of an hour after applying the lymph tape there is already an alleviation of the pain and an increase in the range of movement to dorsal flexion.

5.5.7 Ankle fracture with threatening dystrophy 1st stage, case 7

Case description:

A 57 year old man has fractured his right ankle in a fall. This is not identified in the first instance, only after a week was he referred for an X-ray photo. There appears to be a simple, dislocated, distal tibia fracture which is reduced in an operation and fixed with a plate. This is followed by an immobilisation period with plaster of a total of 7 weeks. This period lasts four weeks longer than planned, because at a check-up too little callus formation is found to be present.
At a check-up three days before the first physiotherapy treatment, there then seems to be sufficient callus formation and he is gradually allowed to exercise and weight bear without plaster.

At the first treatment a clear swelling is visible around the ankle and in the forefoot, the lower leg is slightly swollen. The skin has a red and smooth-shiny appearance particularly around the ankle and in the foot. When not weight-bearing there is no pain present, when weight-bearing there is however pain around the ankle. Upon examination the range of movement of the top and bottom ankle joint is found to be limited and painful in all directions.

During the first treatment the prevention of a dystrophic process should be given priority. An extensive lymph tape is applied, combined with a limited orthopaedic tape for support.

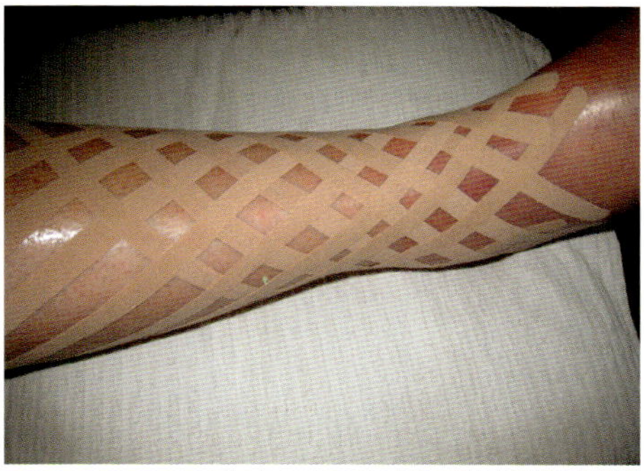

Crossing lymph strips from the popliteal region to just past the ankle; 1st treatment.
Width of the lymph strips: here ± 1.25 cm (5 cm wide tape cut into 4 strips).

Already at the second treatment the red and smooth-shiny appearance of the skin has reasonably returned to normal. Further treatment is given with the same extensive lymph tape construction, at the same time the treatment with orthopaedic tapes is further extended.

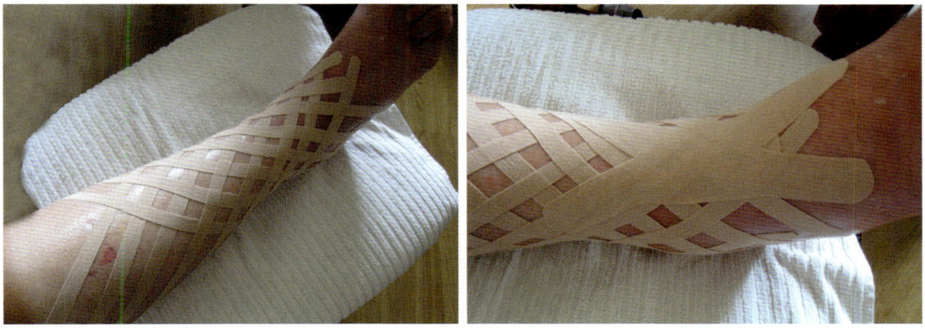

Crossing lymph strips from the popliteal region to just past the ankle; 2nd treatment; here combined with an X-tape level with the retinaculum.
Width of the lymph strips: here ± 1.25 cm (5 cm wide tape cut into 4 strips).

As first orthopaedic tape an X-tape is used as described in § 5.5.2. The X-tape level with the retinaculum serves to give a little more space for the nerves and blood vessels to the forefoot.
After this the stabilising orthopaedic tape is built up further.

After four treatments the client has recovered so far that he can again make long car journeys. He goes off on holiday, the treatment series is completed.

5.5.8 Hallux valgus, post operative, case 5

Case description:

A participant in a course was operated on around four weeks ago for a hallux valgus. It has healed well, but around the operation site there is still a moderate swelling present. During the natural rolling movement of the foot, which is known as foot gait, the joint felt stiff and rigid.

The assumption is that the hard and stiff feeling upon exercise is mainly caused by the swelling present. A lymph tape is therefore constructed from the lower leg.

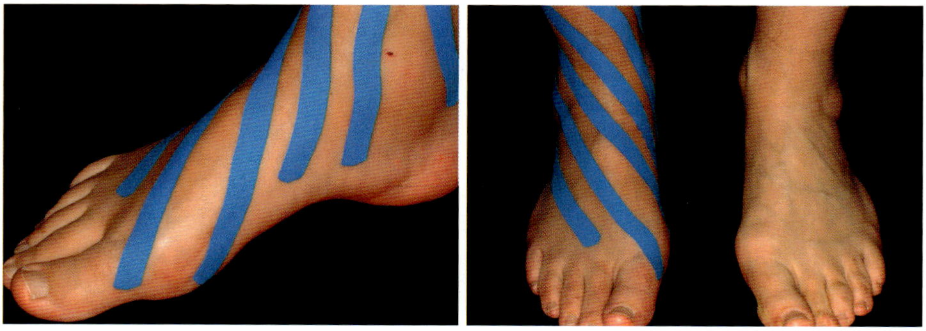

Parallel lymph strips from the lower leg to the forefoot.
Width of the lymph strips: here ± 1.25 cm (5 cm wide tape cut into 4 strips).

Because this involves not too great a problem in someone without underlying complicating factors, it is decided to use a moderately intensive lymph tape. The tape is constructed from half way up the lower leg. It is decided to use parallel lymph strips, not a construction with crossing lymph strips.

After a few hours the participant reported that she felt the rolling movement of her foot to be much more fluid.

5.6 Pregnancy, case 15

Case description:

A 36 year old, pregnant woman comes into the practice because of lymph problems. It is her second pregnancy and she is now in the 13th week. During the first pregnancy four years ago she developed a serious fluid problem, from which she has only slowly recovered after the birth.

During this pregnancy she would like to avoid these problems and comes into the practice with the question of whether this is possible. The pelvic instability symptoms that she suffered during the first pregnancy are already beginning to develop.

Both legs have clearly increased in size, both hands are enlarged. Stemmer's test is positive in the toes and fingers.
The stimulation of lymph drainage from the pelvic area and from the legs in this case has priority. Because of the pregnancy it is decided to construct a lymph tape from central.

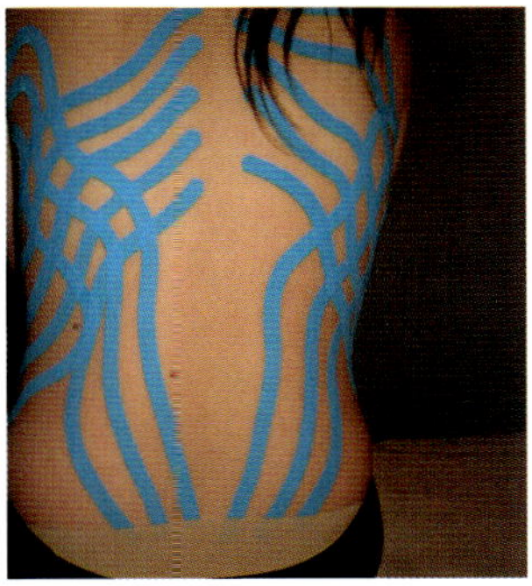

Homolateral lymph strips from axillary to the SI joints combined with homolateral lymph strips from paravertebral to the lateral side of the abdomen. Combination with an orthopaedic tape because of the pelvic instability.
Width of the lymph strips: here ± 1.25 cm (5 cm wide tape cut into 4 strips).

Homolateral, parallel lymph strips from axillary to the SI joints are positioned to prevent fluid accumulation around the pelvic joints. The feeling is that this fluid accumulation partly causes the pelvic instability symptoms.

Furthermore homolateral, parallel lymph strips are positioned from paravertebral to the lateral side of the abdomen. Because of the pregnancy it is decided to tape conservatively, only from central, and not to run the lymph strips further than the abdomen.
This tape is combined with an orthopaedic tape to prevent pelvic instability.

This treatment produces the required effect. In the days after the treatment both legs decrease in size and the pelvic instability symptoms are reduced. Remarkably enough there is also a volume reduction in the hands.

In the course of the pregnancy regular treatment is given. Initially with a low frequency, 1 treatment every 3 to 4 weeks, towards the end of the pregnancy weekly.

As the pregnancy progresses, the lymph tape construction is extended further, although the tapes remain central.

The extension consists of extra tapes being positioned from homolateral cervical paravertebral to the M. Trapezius and M. Deltoideus region. From homolateral lumbar paravertebral a pair of extra lymph strips are applied to the gluteal region.

Although the symptoms increase in the course of the pregnancy, as expected, the opinion of the client is that the symptoms are increasing much less than during the first pregnancy.

Six months after starting the treatment a healthy son is born.

5.7 Haematomas, fibroses and scars

5.7.1 Haematomas, local swellings and fibroses

The increased tissue pressure that occurs in case of haematomas or local swellings can be treated with a more or less extensive lymph tape construction.

If there are no circumstances which are already putting an extra load on the lymphatic system, a local crossed lymph tape will usually suffice. If there are additional taxing circumstances, which is a reason to choose a more intensive treatment with longer lymph strips from a more proximal located drainage area. Factors that produce an extra load for the drainage of local swellings or haematomas include:

- Medication, for example blood-thinning medication;
- Heart trouble;
- Kidney trouble;
- Underlying pathology such as primary or secondary lymphoedema (see chapters 6 and 7);
- Very extensive and/or several sites with swellings or haematomas.

Here only one example of local treatment is shown. The structure of the treatment is similar to the description in § 5.5.2., for more treatment examples please refer to this paragraph.

The area to be treated is amply covered with lymph strips. In the case of haematomas or swellings of limited size, taping is not peripheral to the treatment area. However, with a more substantial swelling or haematoma, part of this will move in the interstitial tissue to peripheral. If it is expected that this may happen, that is a reason to still have the lymph strips run slightly further to peripheral.

By applying the lymph strips of the grid from proximal to peripheral, the treatment emphasis lies in the direction of the lymph flow.

If it is not possible to stretch the skin due to the starting position, the skin can be stretched more by moving it more to proximal with the hand.

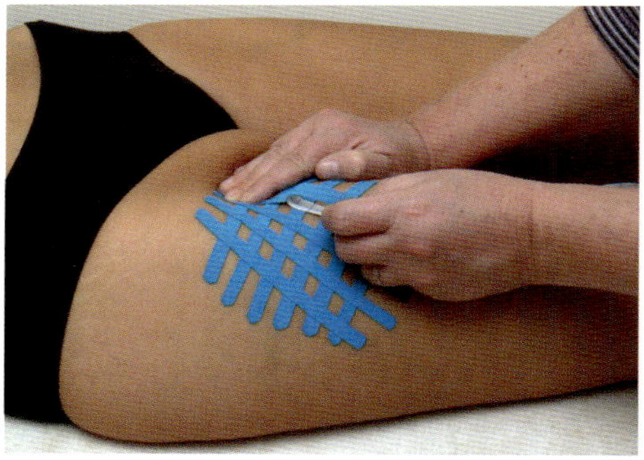
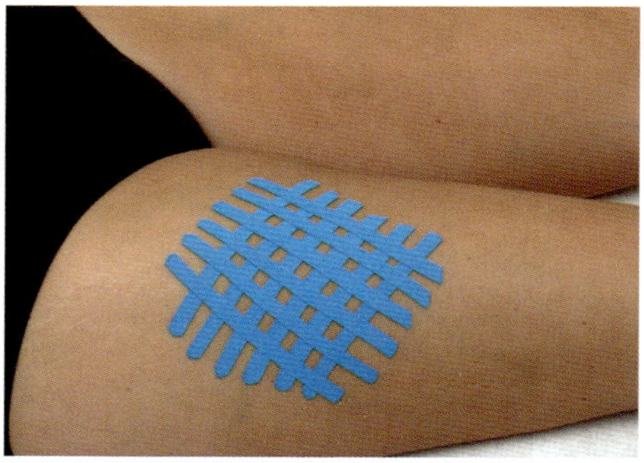

Crossed local lymph strips, applied from proximal to peripheral.
Width of the lymph strips: here ± 1 cm (5 cm wide tape cut into 5 strips).

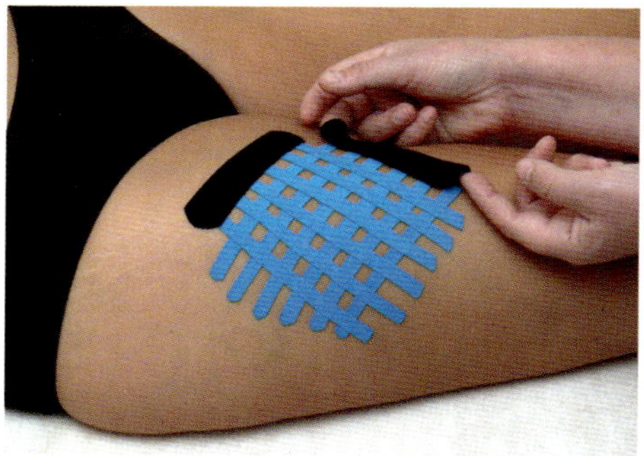
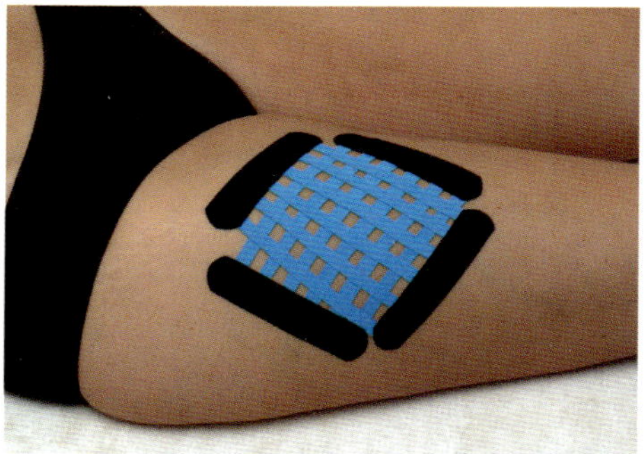

With blue tape here the working lymph strips are applied, with the black tape strips the anchors are reinforced. The black tape is not active tape and so is applied without stretch in the skin or tape.

The anchors of the narrow lymph strips can be covered with a wider tape strip, so that the total tape construction can remain in place better and for longer. The only function of the wider CureTape strip is reinforcement of the lymph strips, and is therefore applied without stretch in the skin or tape. Also the 10% pretensioning of the tape is eliminated.

In the case of fibrotic tissue the same technique can be used, the lymph strips are in that case however applied with a little more stretch. The basic principle is: the harder the tissue to be treated, the more stretch must be put in the working tape strips.

5.7.2 Haematoma, case 32

Case description:
A 24 year old nurse who is under treatment in the practice for primary lymphoedema states during the treatment that she is bothered by a haematoma. The treatment consists of manual lymph drainage, an exercise schedule and rules for life. During her work she wears support tights, pressure class 2. This keeps the lymphoedema under good control and at the moment stable.

The haematoma is indeed limited in size, but because of the underlying lymph problems is expected to drain slowly. The haematoma is therefore treated with CureTape. The tape treatment is a little more intensive than a local crossed lymph tape. From proximal slightly longer lymph strips are used that cross over one another in the haematoma area.

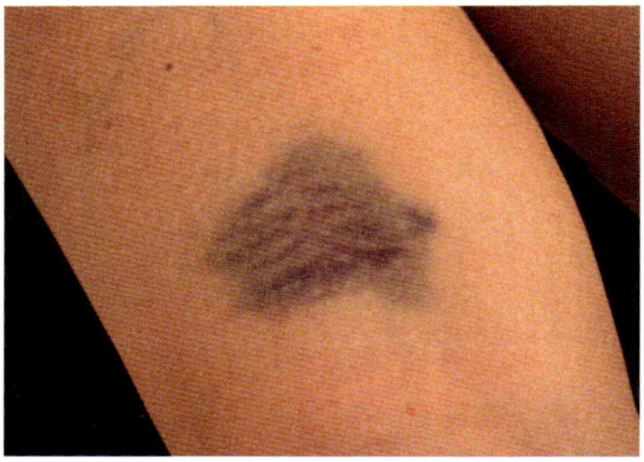

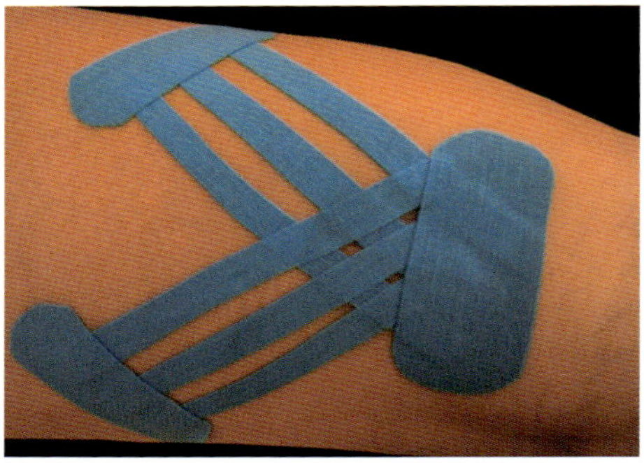

Slightly longer lymph strips from proximal, crossing in the haematoma area. With the slightly wider tape strips the anchors are additionally reinforced.
Width of the lymph strips: here ± 1.25 cm (5 cm wide tape cut into 4 strips).

This tape treatment was found to be sufficient and did not have to be repeated.

5.7.3 Trauma with haematoma, case 2

Case description:
A 76 year old man has fallen off his bicycle and has thereby suffered a considerable haematoma in his left leg, with an open wound on the medial side of the lower leg. The recovery is going very slowly, partly because of the use of blood-thinning medication. Weight-bearing is poor because of the pain, the inactivity is also delaying the recovery.
He hears of the possibilities with Medical Taping and therefore two weeks after the accident comes into the practice for treatment. The haematoma is at that time in particular visible around the ankle and in the foot, also on the back of the knee. The wound on the lower leg is still not fully closed, around the wound a considerable swelling is present.

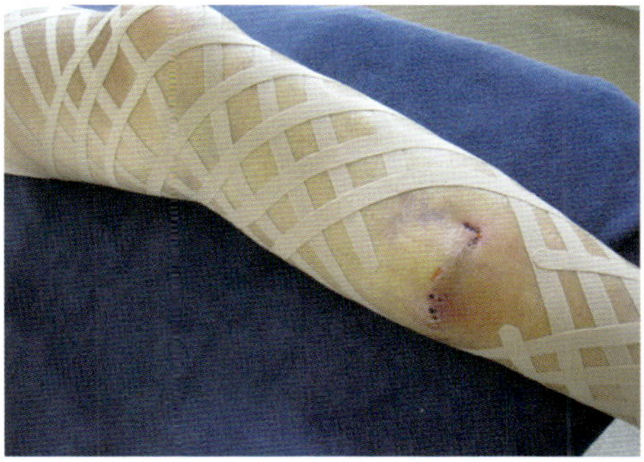
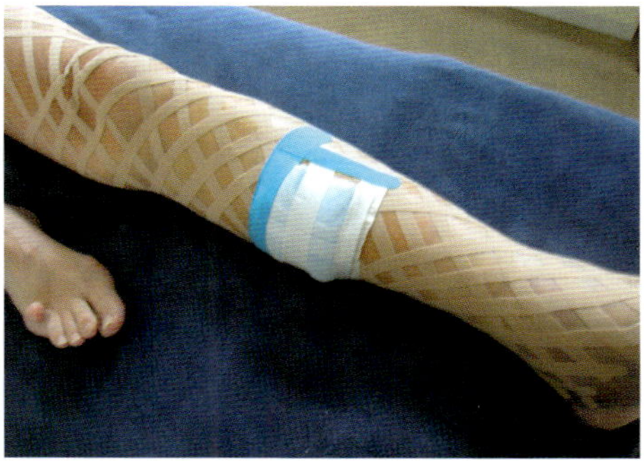

Parallel lymph strips from the lower abdomen to the foot. The wound area remains free to make wound care possible. The treatment emphasis lies in the distal part. Width of the lymph strips: here ± 1.25 cm (5 cm wide tape cut into 4 strips).

Because the wound has not yet fully closed it is not possible to tape over this area, furthermore wound care should remain possible. The considerable swelling around the wound area would under other circumstances be a reason not to tape peripheral from the wound, as after all this would conduct lymph fluid into the problem area. There is however also a considerable haematoma here around the ankle and in the foot, so it is decided in this case to still apply the lymph strips to the foot.

Because of the extent of the problem and because of the medication, lymph tape treatment is constructed with longer lymph strips which are applied from the lower abdomen to the foot. Here it is ensured that the wound area remains free of tape.
In the upper leg the space between the lymph strips is slightly greater, more towards the lower leg the space between the lymph strips is clearly narrower. In this way the treatment emphasis lies in the lower leg, the area where the problem is mainly located.
After a week at the second treatment the effect of the lymph tape is already clearly visible. The pain present has gradually reduced during the first treatment week, so the activity level has gradually increased. The client is now walking two to three kilometres a day and has also been cycling again.

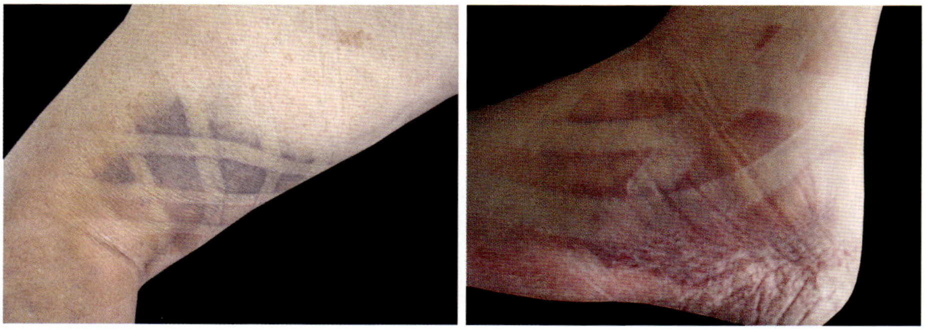

Detailed photos of the effect of the first treatment with lymph taping. Under the lymph strips the haematoma has already greatly reduced, so the outline of the tape strips is visible.

At the second treatment the skin over the wound is found to be partly closed, in part there is still a scab present. Tape can be applied over the closed skin, the scab is not covered with tape.
Because the swelling around the wound has only moderately reduced, the treatment emphasis of the second treatment lies around this area. A local grid is made with narrow lymph strips, after which longer lymph strips are applied from the lower abdomen which end around the swollen wound area.

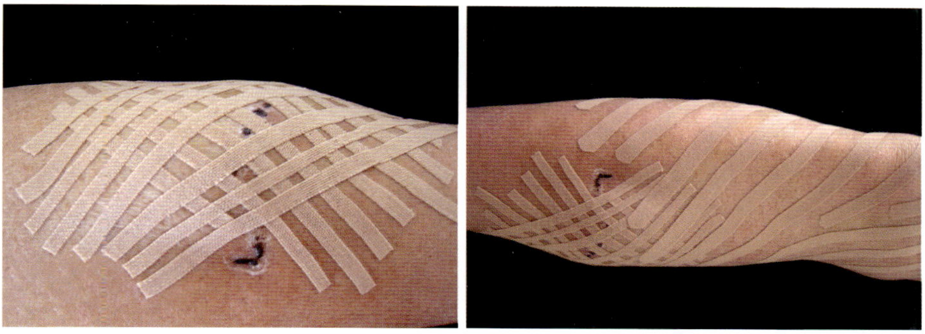

Local narrow crossed lymph strips. Slightly wider parallel lymph strips applied from the lower abdomen end in the area around the wound.
Width of the tape: the local crossed lymph strips are ± 0.6 cm wide (5 cm wide tape cut into 8 strips). The longer parallel lymph strips are ± 1.25 cm wide (5 cm wide tape cut into 4 strips).

After this a third treatment is carried out. The situation has by then already improved so much that a fourth treatment is no longer necessary.

The effect of lymph taping is most clearly visible in the treatment of a haematoma. When the tape is removed after a few days, the lymph strips are outlined in the haematoma. Under the lymph strips a large proportion of the haematoma has already drained, in the skin area located between the lymph strips the haematoma is still much more present.

From this the conclusion could be drawn that the effect of the tape would be even better if the whole haematoma was covered with tape. This is however not the case, the action of a lymph tape is better if narrow strips are used (see also § 4.6.2).

Furthermore the conclusion could be drawn, that at the second treatment the lymph strips should be positioned exactly over the visible remains of the haematoma. This can be difficult to achieve and is also not really worth it, because the lymph strips ensure improved drainage as a result of which the remains of the haematoma will as it were be 'absorbed'.

5.7.4 Scars

Both fresh, not yet sealed scars and older and/or sealed scars may be a reason to treat with tape.
By treating a fresh scar with CureTape, the growth of lymph vessels in the area is stimulated. This promotes recovery and at the same time avoids the scar sealing.
The tape is not sterile, therefore in the case of fresh scars tape treatment can only be started when the scar is closed and covered with skin.
The tissue of older and/or sealed scars can be softened by treating with tape. The basic principle is also used here: the harder the tissue to be treated, the more stretch must be put on the working tape strips.

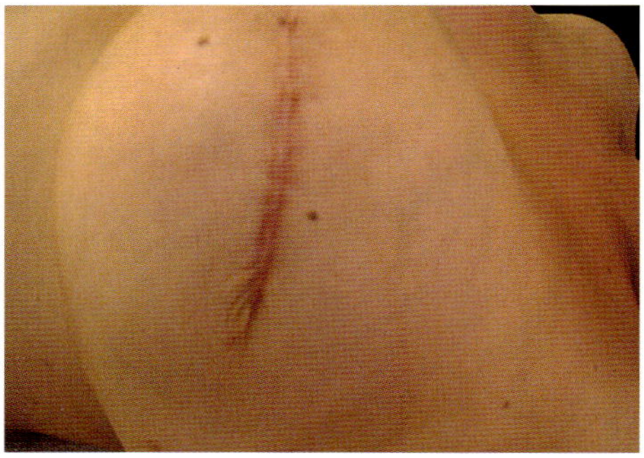

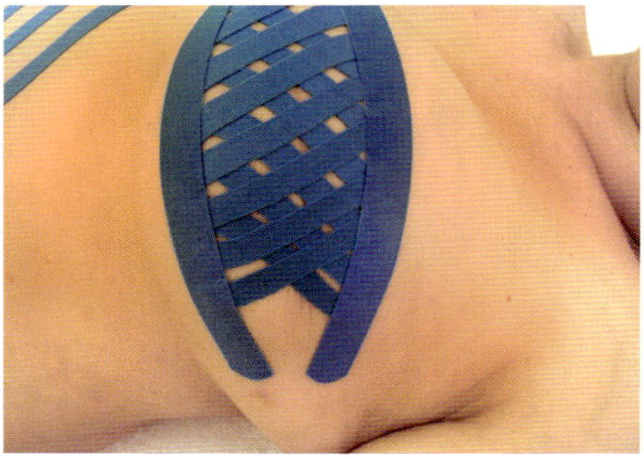

Scar treatment; for a more extensive case description see § 6.3.2.
Width of the tape strips: here ± 1 cm wide (5 cm wide tape cut into 5 strips).

If swelling is present around the scar, it may be decided to apply the tape strips in the direction of the lymph drainage. Because the direction of action of the tape is the opposite to the tape direction, the lymph strips are applied from the drainage area to the treatment area. In this way the scar treatment is combined with lymph tape treatment.
If no swelling is present around the scar, the paper of the tape strip can be torn in the middle, after which the tape strip can be placed over the scar from the middle.

5.7.5 Scar treatment, case 31

Case description:

During a course one of the participants says that she has had a right lower arm fracture, which was treated surgically with osteosynthesis material. In view of the symptoms that the osteosynthesis material produced, this has recently been removed.

The scars have healed well, but the scar tissue is quite hard. The whole lower arm is still rather swollen. Her question is whether tape treatment could help.

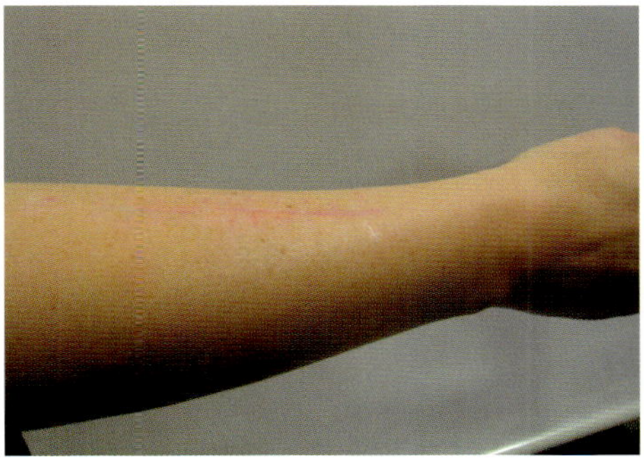

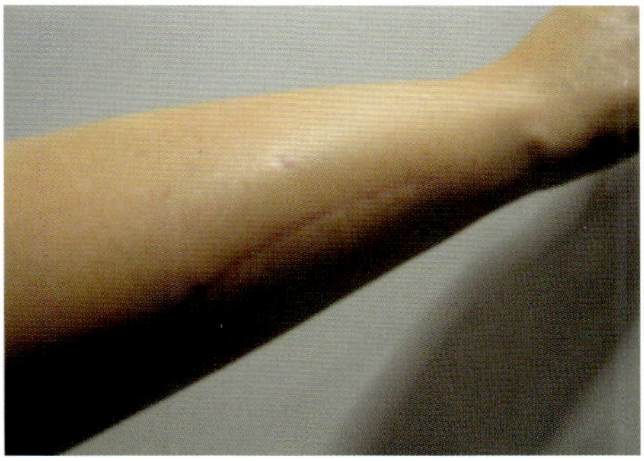

Scars along radius and ulna, with a moderate swelling of the lower arm.

Because of the swelling it is decided to use a parallel lymph tape, applied from the elbow area to distal. Because the scar tissue feels quite hard, the tape strips are applied in the scar area with more stretch in the tape.

The other part of the tape strips is applied as a normal lymph tape that is with stretch in the skin, but without extra stretch in the tape.

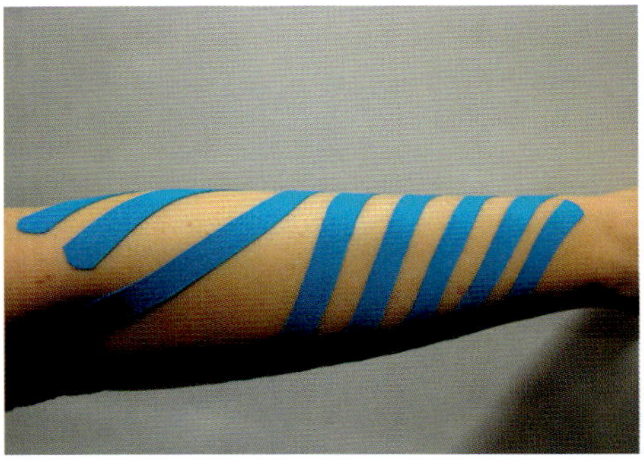
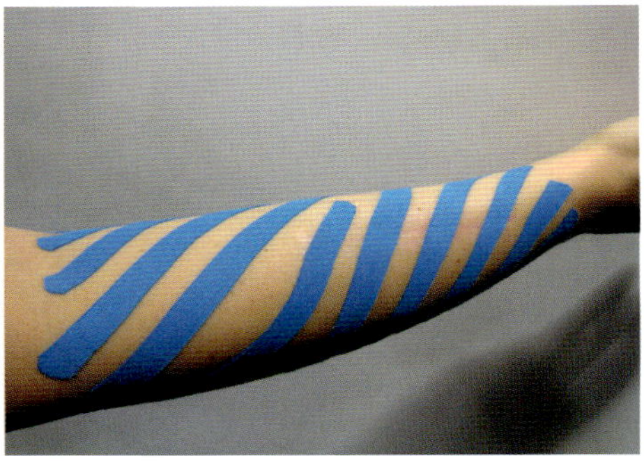

Combined lymph and scar treatment; parallel lymph strips from the elbow to distal, in the scar area applied with extra stretch in the tape.
Width of the tape strips: here ± 1.25 cm (5 cm wide tape cut into 4 strips).

A crossing lymph tape would give a more intensive action, but is not always well tolerated. The extent of the swelling was decisive here for the choice of working with a parallel lymph tape.

As soon as the swelling has disappeared, the scars can be treated with a local crossed tape. The advice to the course member is to continue the scar treatment until the tissue is soft and supple again.

6. Secondary lymphoedema

6.1 Introduction

The occurrence of secondary lymphoedema was discussed in chapter 3. In the treatment of secondary lymphoedema manual lymph drainage remains an important part of the treatment, even if it is decided to use lymph taping in the treatment.
Lymph taping can be used in combination with compression therapy (see § 4.4), where taping is carried out proximal from the stocking or bandage. Parts of the body which cannot or can hardly be treated with compression therapy, can however often be treated using lymph taping, while at the same time compression therapy remains possible for other parts of the body.

It is however also possible to replace the compression therapy by treatment with lymph taping. During the writing of this book there is not yet any valid scientific research available which shows that this method of treatment is more effective than treatment with compression therapy. However various national and international research projects have already been set up in which the interim evaluation can be called promising.

A lot of experience from practice has been acquired since around 1999/2000 with the treatment of secondary lymphoedema, where lymph taping is used as an adjunct to manual lymph drainage. Empirically it may cautiously be stated that the results of this treatment combination are certainly not inferior to the results achieved when using the combination MLD and compression therapy.

The advantages of using lymph taping are evident. A big advantage of treatment with lymph taping is that the tape is felt to be much less stressful than compression therapy. For many clients it means a considerable improvement in their quality of life. Another advantage is that lymph taping can often be used for parts of the body where compression therapy is difficult or impossible. Furthermore with lymph taping it is possible to work much more flexibly with the stimulation of anastomoses (see also § 4.8.2 and § 4.8.3).
It can be seen as a disadvantage that it is not possible for everyone to tape themselves, which means the client would remain dependent on the therapist. In these cases a carer can sometimes offer a solution.

6.2 Lymph taping after radiotherapy

Taping may not be carried out in the radiation area during and directly after radiotherapy. The skin must have recovered sufficiently and be able to withstand strain before this area can be taped.

During this period it is possible to tape *around* the irradiated skin area. When taping around the irradiated area, the lymphatic pressure in this surrounding area will be reduced and the lymph flow from an area with a higher lymphatic pressure will be stimulated. Because the lymphatic system has anastomoses between vessels located more on the surface and those located deeper, lymph drainage from the problem area is also possible along this pathway.

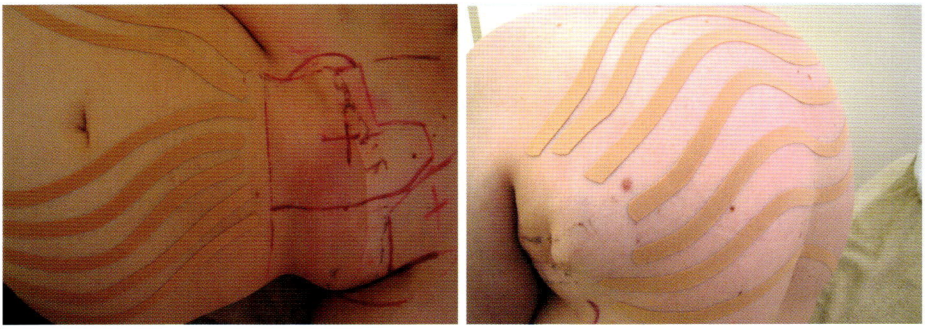

Lymph tape around the radiation area, § 6.3.3, case 34.

It is also not possible to tape round this area in the initial period after irradiation. It is assumed that a minimum recovery period of six weeks is necessary before the irradiated area can be safely taped.

In practice this period varies quite a lot, because many factors may affect the recovery of the skin. The recovery period of six weeks mentioned sometimes seems rather generous, but in some cases the recovery period may even be twice as long.

If tape treatment is started too early, this will certainly cause skin damage and hence have negative consequences on the lymphatic pressure.

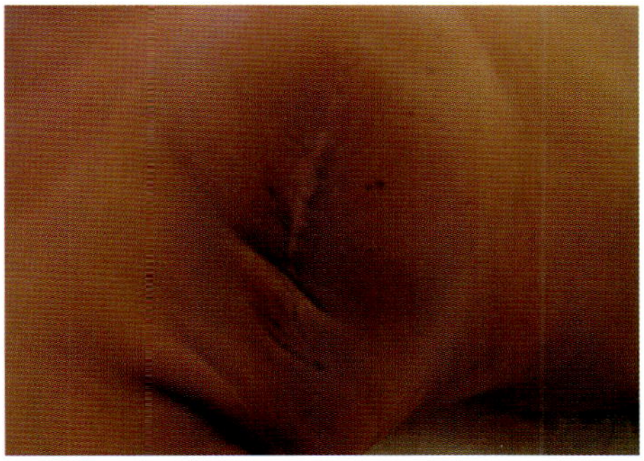

Skin with effect of radiotherapy, four weeks after the end of irradiation; § 6.3.2, case 20.

When the skin seems to have recovered sufficiently, in consultation with the client an attempt can be made to apply a small piece of lymph tape to the irradiation area. If after a few days this is found not to have caused any problems, the treatment can then gradually be extended further.

6.3 Axillary node dissection

After a partial or total mastectomy where the axillary lymph nodes have also been removed, lymph congestion may occur in all areas that normally drain via the armpit. Lymphoedema may develop in the homolateral arm, the breast and the flank.

Because alternative drainage paths are possible, the problem of the lymph congestion does not have to occur. But the chance that lymphoedema will occur continues to exist for the rest of the life, even if there have been no symptoms for years after the procedure.

Immediately after the operation the scar forms an extra obstruction to lymph drainage, the surface lymph vessels are cut through and have not yet regenerated. The effects of the irradiation may further obstruct lymph drainage. Once the scar is closed with skin, a start can be made with the tape treatment, taking into account the restrictions that radiotherapy can cause (see also § 5.7.4 and § 6.2). Before the scar is fully closed, it is however possible to tape around the scar.

Because there is a functional restriction of the natural drainage path, it is natural during the treatment to choose a tape construction with anastomoses. The choice can be made of different anastomoses or combinations of these.

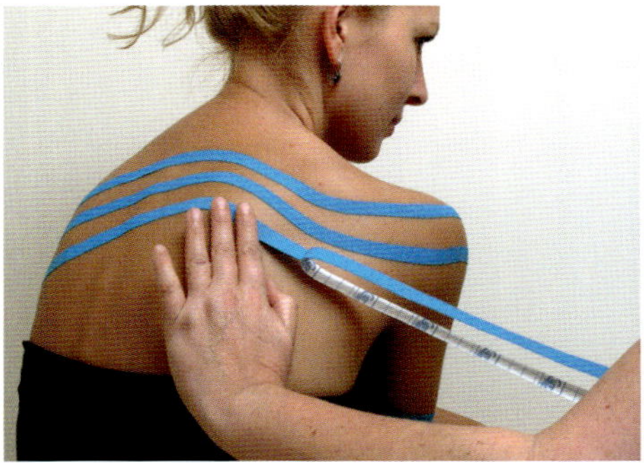

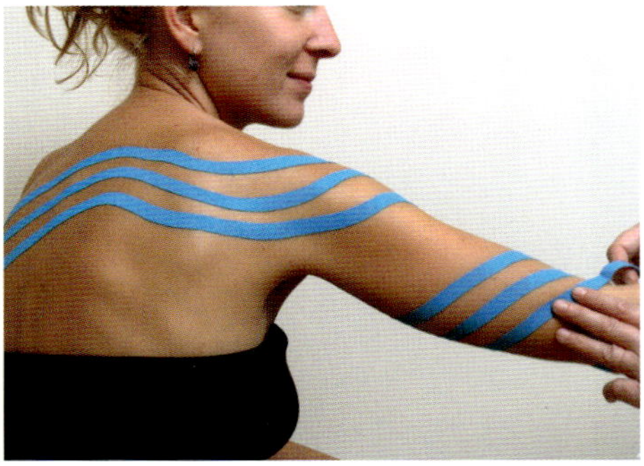

Parallel lymph strips from heterolateral axillary to the arm.
Width of the lymph strips: here ± 1.25 cm (5 cm wide tape cut into 4 strips.

Here a lymph tape is shown that is constructed from the heterolateral axillary area. The lymph strips can be applied to the arm without interruption. Depending on the problem and the phase of the treatment, the strips can run more or less far into the arm.
The strips remain proximal from the area with lymph congestion or end in this area, but taping is never carried out distal from the problem. If the hand also has to be treated, the lymph strips end in the wrist crease. The hand is taped separately (see also § 5.4.8).
The armpit can be delimited with lymph strips. Lymph strips that run through the armpit will work loose much sooner. If no more anastomosis strips pass over the shoulder while more strips are necessary for the arm, then the extra strips can be 'attached' to one of the previous strips. In this way a spread continues to exist.

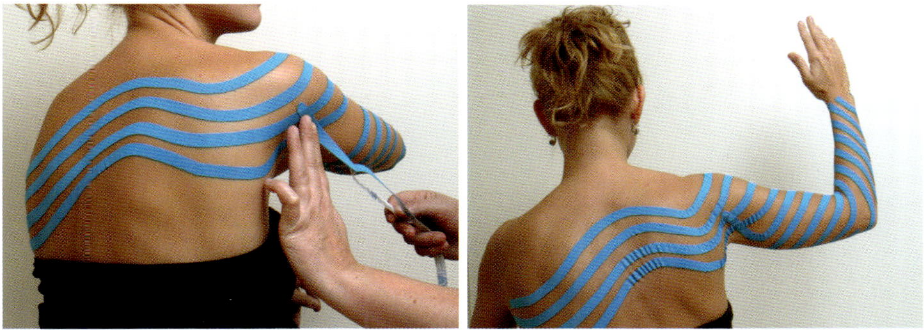

Parallel lymph strips from heterolateral axillary to the arm, with a strip that is 'attached' level with the shoulder.
Width of the lymph strips: here ± 1.25 cm (5 cm wide tape cut into 4 strips)

The treatment with parallel lymph strips can be made more intensive, by constructing extra anastomoses from another drainage area, which cross the first lymph strips.
For these crossing lymph strips, the supraclavicular drainage area on the heterolateral side is used here, where the strips run along the ventral.
By taping the crossing lymph strips along the ventral, a concentration of lymph strips on the dorsal side is avoided.

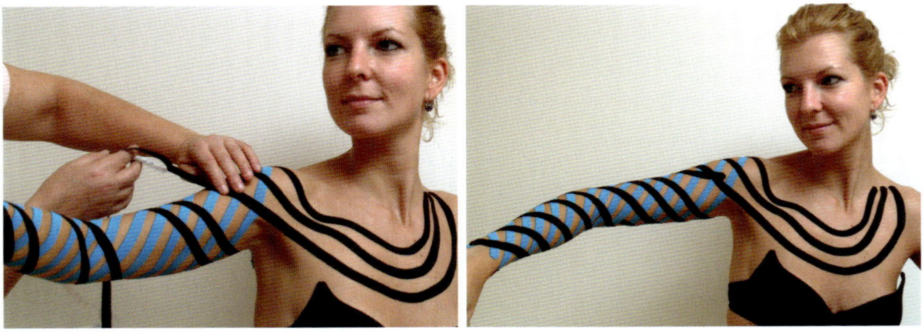

Crossing parallel lymph strips from heterolateral supraclavicular, applied ventrally.
Width of the lymph strips: here around 1.25 cm (5 cm wide tape cut into 4 strips).

With the previous tape construction the lymphoedema in the arm is treated. If there is also lymphoedema in the flank, the tape treatment can be extended. From another drainage area lymph strips can be applied to the oedema in the flank, so that here too the lymph drainage is further stimulated.

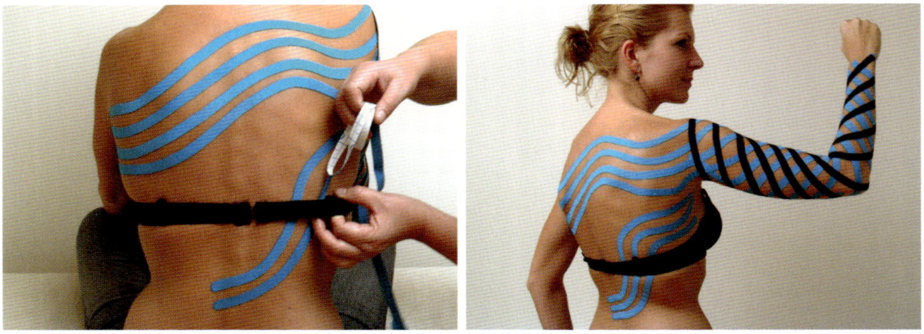

Tape similar to the above discription, supplemented with lymph strips from hetero-lateral paravertebral lumbar to the oedema in the flank.
Width of the lymph strips: here ± 1.25 cm (5 cm wide tape cut into 4 strips).

Also if it is necessary to tape the hand, the lymph strips over the arm end level with the wrist crease. As described in § 5.4.8 the hand usually forms an exception in lymph taping and the tape is applied to the back of the hand from distal to proximal. For an extensive description of the possibilities for a lymph tape on the hand, please refer to § 5.4.8

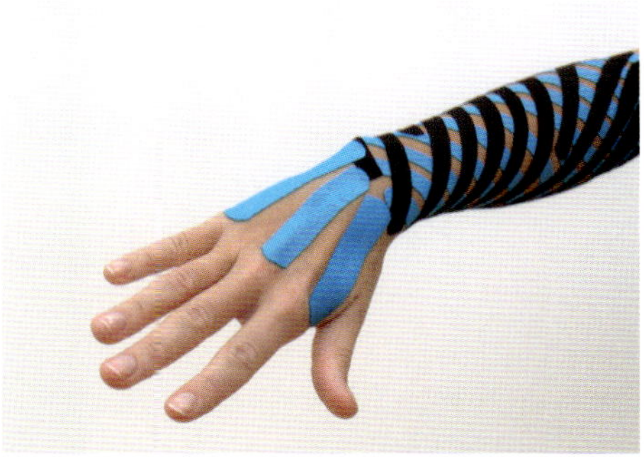

Intensive crossed lymph tape for the arm, supplemented with a hand tape.
Width of the lymph strips: on the arm ± 1.25 cm (5 cm wide tape cut into 4 strips), for the hand ± 1.65 cm wide (5 cm wide tape cut into 3 strips).

If there is a reason to extend the tape treatment to the fingers as well then that can be done with a tape construction as shown and described in § 5.4.9. The fingers drain in the direction of the hand, so on the fingers the lymph strips are again applied from proximal to distal.

Note: in practice it regularly happens that carpal tunnel syndrome is diagnosed after a homolateral lymph node resection. Also if there is no visible, measureable or palpable oedema, the symptoms usually disappear as soon as treatment with manual lymph drainage and lymph taping is started. Operative procedures may in these cases cause a latent lymphoedema present to become manifest.

6.3.1 Axillary node dissection, case 4

Case description:
A 62 year old nurse comes into the practice, six months after breast cancer has been confirmed for the second time. The first breast cancer was on the left side and was treated around a year and a half ago with a breast-conserving operation, without lymph node resection.

Six months ago breast cancer was confirmed on the right side. This treatment also consisted of a breast-conserving operation, but with an axillary node dissection.
Both times the follow-up treatment has consisted of radiotherapy, both times she has had no chemotherapy.
She has no symptoms on the left side. Recently however symptoms have occurred on the right side, particularly in the right breast there is a palpable and visible lymphoedema present. The tissue around the scar also feels rather hard.

There is no perceptible, visible or measurable difference in size in the arms. She does however sometimes experience pressure in the right M. Deltoideus region if her activity level has been higher than normal. Some pressure may then also occur in the flank.
Furthermore she has regular neck complaints and there is a slight movement restriction in the anteflexion direction on the right side that has already been present for a few years after suffering bursitis. The shoulder has not caused any further problems in recent years.

Manual lymph drainage was started, supplemented with a CureTape treatment. Initially the tape treatment was limited, because the manual treatment is also still being built up (see also § 4.8.2). At the first treatment an anastomosis was taped from lumbar heterolateral paravertebral to the side of the right breast with only three lymph strips. This tape treatment is gradually being extended, until at the fourth treatment the following lymph tapes are applied.

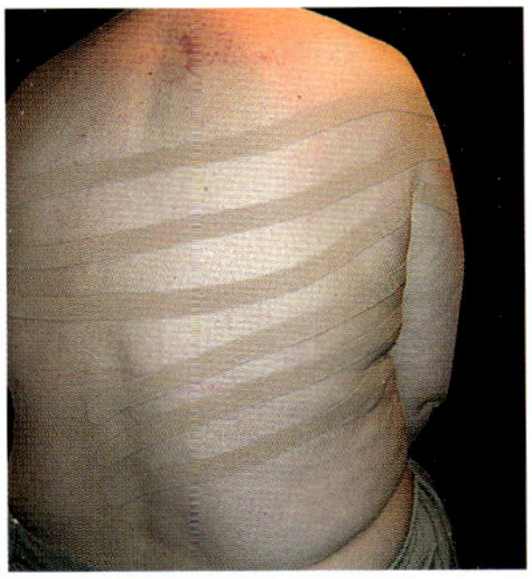

Three lymph strips from lumbar heterolateral paravertebral ending at the fibrosis tape on the lateral side of the breast; three lymph strips from the heterolateral axillary region via dorsal ending in the deltoid region.
Width of the lymph strips: here ±1.25 cm (5 cm wide tape cut into 4 strips).

- Crossed fibrosis tape over the scar, because of the hardness of the tissue applied with around ¾ of the maximum stretch;
- Three lymph strips from heterolateral lumbar via the flank to the lateral side of the breast;
- Three lymph strips from homolateral inguinal to the caudal side of the breast;
- Three lymph strips from the heterolateral inguinal to the medial side of the breast;
- Two lymph strips from heterolateral supraclavicular via the ventral side to the craniomedial side of the right breast;
- Three lymph strips from heterolateral axillary via the mid-thoracic spine to the right deltoid region.

By combining these different anastomosis tapes with one another, an attempt is made to spread the lymph drainage as far as possible and to create as big as possible a reabsorption area.

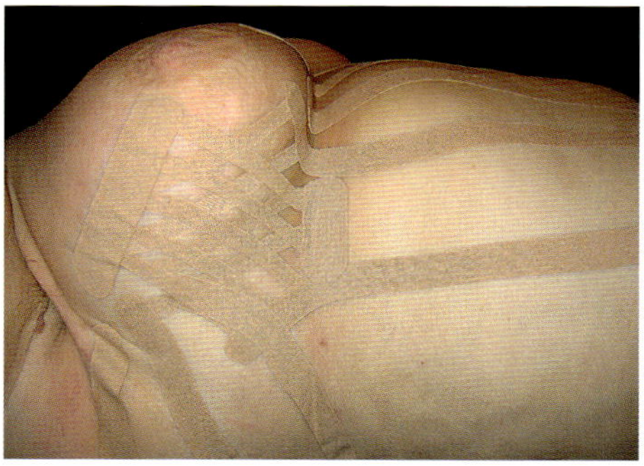

Fibrosis tape over the scar; three lymph strips from lumbar heterolateral paravertebral ending lateral from the fibrosis tape; three lymph strips from homolateral inguinal to the caudal side of the breast; three lymph strips from heterolateral inguinal ending on the medial side of the breast.

Width of the lymph strips: here ± 1.25 cm (5 cm wide tape cut into 4 strips); width of the lymph strips over the scar: here ± 0.6 cm (5 cm wide tape cut into 8 strips). The ends of the fibrosis tape are additionally reinforced with 2½ cm wide tape to prevent it working loose prematurely.

The regularly returning neck symptoms are the reason to avoid the cervicothoracic area with lymph tape. As a result it is not really possible to apply an anastomosis tape from heterolateral supraclavicular via the dorsal side.

After having done one treatment in this way, it is found at the next treatment that a volume increase has occurred in the left breast. Because of the risk of a so-called 'overflow oedema', the anastomosis is therefore no longer used from heterolateral supraclavicular.

A further four treatments follow in which the tapes mentioned are used, with exception of the anastomosis from heterolateral supraclavicular. The situation improves during this time, the oedema in the breast is reduced and the tissue around the scar gradually becomes more supple.

The deltoid region and the flank still only cause trouble sometimes in case of a clearly increased activity level, but that disappears spontaneously again within 24 to 48 hours.

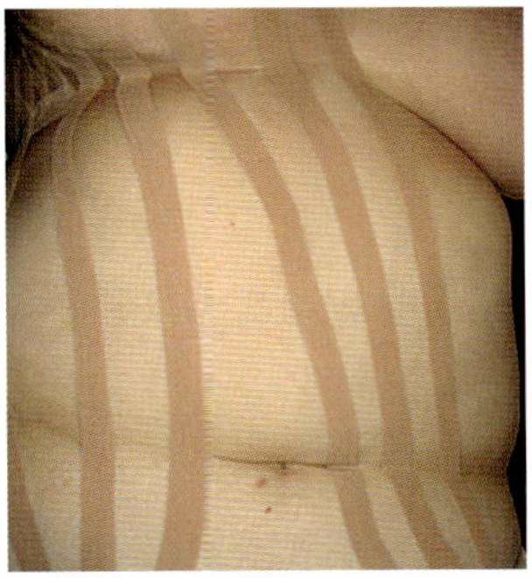

Three lymph strips from homolateral inguinal to the caudal side of the breast; three lymph strips from heterolateral inguinal ending on the medial side of the breast.
Width of the lymph strips: here around 1.25 cm (5 cm wide tape cut into 4 strips).

After these four treatments the lymph strips applied from inguinal to the underside of the breast appear to cause a few infection sites on the underside of the breast. The cotton on the tape remains slightly damp after showering which is causing this problem.

Hence it is also no longer possible to use the anastomosis tapes from inguinal. There are then only two possibilities for anastomosis tapes left. The first possibility is from paravertebral, at levels caudal from mid-thoracic. The second possibility is from heterolateral axillary, along the dorsal side.

Because of the improved situation that is enough. The frequency of the treatment is then already reduced to one treatment every two weeks. Because of a house move the treatment was then transferred.

6.3.2 Axillary node dissection, case 20

Case description:

A 39 year old manager comes into the practice with lymphoedema in the breast. Around six months before breast cancer was confirmed in the right breast. In view of the size of the tumour the treatment was started with chemotherapy.

Four months after starting chemotherapy a mastectomy is carried out with axillary node dissection on the right side. The left breast is removed at the same time as a precaution. During the operation temporary implants are fitted on both sides for the breast reconstruction that will follow.

When she comes into the practice for treatment, the temporary implants are still being gradually topped up weekly. In the right breast considerable engorgement has occurred, which was aspirated a few days ago. Although during this aspiration a litre and a half of fluid was removed, there is still considerable lymph congestion.

There is no measurable, visible or palpable difference in the size of the arms, she has however a rather dragging feeling in the right armpit. In the right shoulder there is a slight restriction in the anteflexion/exorotation direction. There are no problems on the left side.

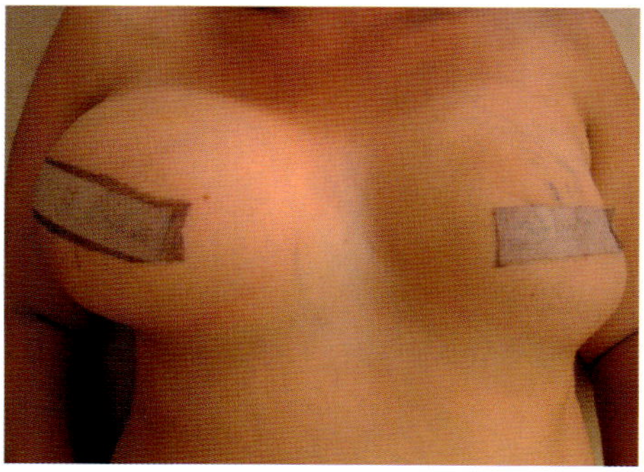

Situation at the start of the first lymph treatment.

The first treatment is started with manual lymph drainage, supplemented with limited tape treatment. The lymph tape is applied on the dorsal side with two strips from heterolateral supraclavicular and two strips heterolateral axillary, ending on the lateral side of the right breast.

On the ventral side four lymph strips are applied from heterolateral inguinal, ending on the caudal side and the medial side of the right breast.

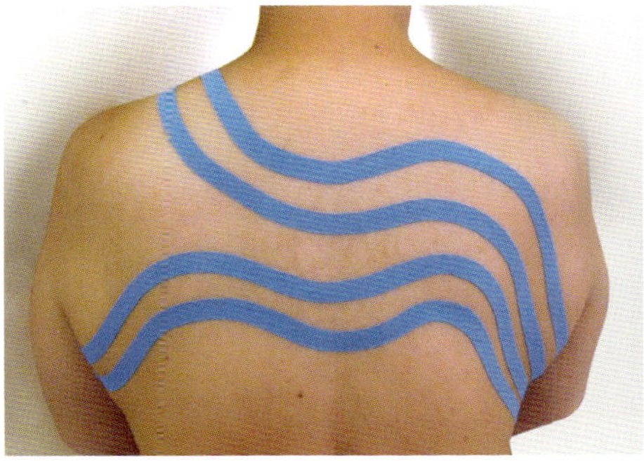
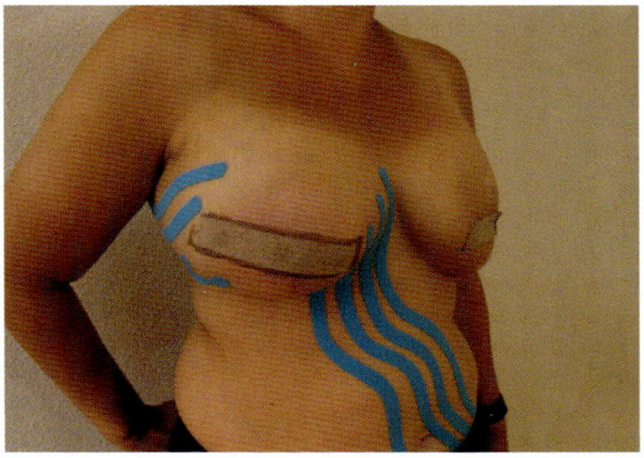

First treatment: two lymph strips from heterolateral supraclavicular and two lymph strips from heterolateral axillary, via the dorsal side ending on the lateral side of the breast; four lymph strips from heterolateral inguinal ending on the caudal and the medial side of the breast.
Width of the lymph strips: here around 1.25 cm (5 cm wide tape cut into 4 strips).

By making anastomoses with the lymph tape from three different areas, an attempt is made to spread the lymph drainage as far as possible and to increase the reabsorption area.

Three days after this treatment in the hospital a further ¾ litre of fluid is removed. She herself has the feeling that the build up of lymph congestion is clearly less than the week preceding the first treatment. There is however still a substantial lymphoedema present in the right breast.

At the second treatment the manual lymph drainage is supplemented with a rather more extensive lymph tape. Apart from the dorsal strips, two lymph strips are now also applied from homolateral supraclavicular to the cranial side of the breast. In addition three extra lymph strips are applied from homolateral inguinal to the caudal side of the breast.

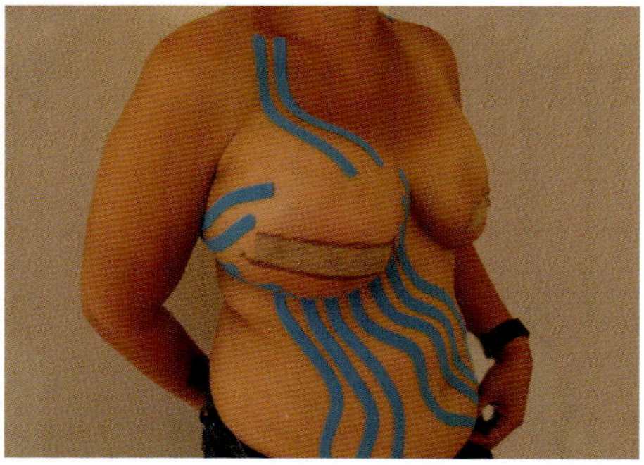

Second treatment: two lymph strips from heterolateral supraclavicular and two lymph strips from heterolateral axillary, via the dorsal side ending on the lateral side of the breast; two lymph strips from homolateral supraclavicular ending on the cranial side of the breast; four lymph strips from heterolateral inguinal ending on the caudal and the medial side of the breast; three lymph strips from homolateral inguinal ending on the caudal side of the breast.
Width of the lymph strips: here ± 1.25 cm (5 cm wide tape cut into 4 strips.

Because the treatment has only just started, the tape strips are not yet applied further into the breast but end everywhere just in the oedema area. If the lymph drainage is stimulated from the edges of the breast, the lymphatic pressure in these areas will become lower, as a result of which the lymph can be drained from the breast better.

Three days after this treatment a further 120 ml is removed in the hospital. The lymphoedema in the breast begins to clearly reduce anc after this no further aspiration will be carried out.

At the third treatment the lymph tapes from homolateral supraclavicular appear to have already worked loose within two days after application. During manual lymph drainage the homolateral supraclavicular area also feels overfull. Lymph strips from this area therefore seem to be able to add little.

The adhesive plaster has meanwhile been removed from the scars, so a start can be made with CureTape treatment for the scars. Because the radiotherapy will start within the foreseeable future, only the scar on the left breast is taped. For the right breast no risks of avoidable skin damage may be taken. However taping may be carried out around the irradiation area.

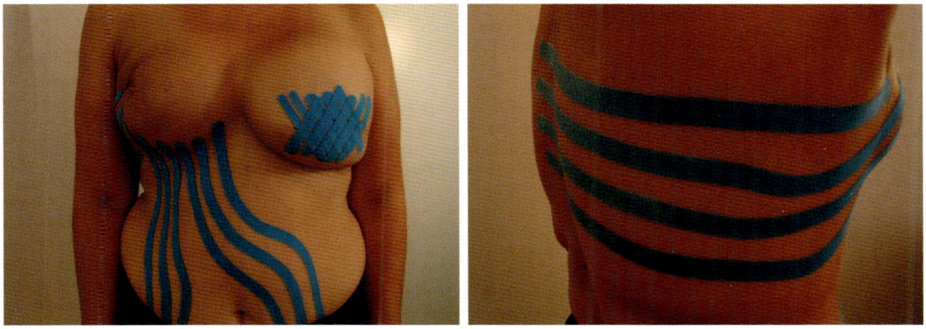

Third treatment: crossed scar tape on the left breast; right four lymph strips from heterolateral axillary to the lateral side of the breast, three lymph strips from heterolateral inguinal and three lymph strips from homolateral inguinal to the caudal side of the breast.

Width of the lymph strips: here ± 1.25 cm (5 cm wide tape cut into 4 strips).

The volume increase that can be seen in the photo of the third treatment is caused in the left breast because the temporary implants are still being gradually topped up. This is also being done on the right side.

Subsequently however part of the filling in the left breast has to be removed again, because the volume was found to obstruct the irradiation. After the radiotherapy this was replaced again. This is the explanation for the volume changes in the left breast as can be seen in the follow-up photos

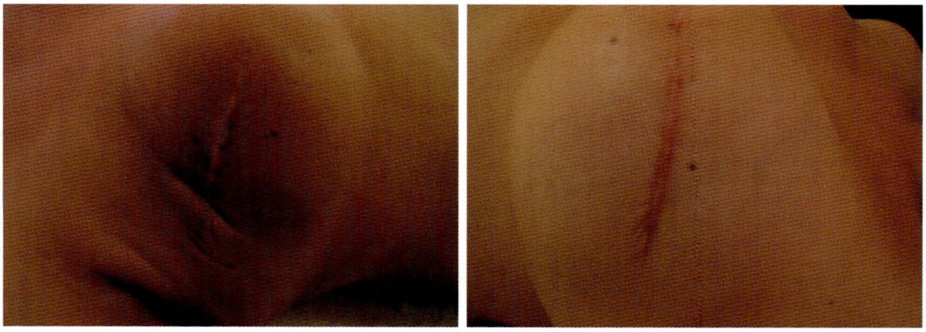

Scars of the right breast and the left breast, the skin of the right breast shows the effect of the radiotherapy.

In the period during and after the irradiation the treatment continues to consist of manual lymph drainage supplemented with tape treatment similar to the third treatment. The lymph strips are then a bit shorter and remain outside the irradiation area.

The skin has remained healthy during the radiotherapy and also recovers well after the radiotherapy. Five weeks after ending the radiotherapy the skin appears to be well recovered and can withstand strain. In the treatment an attempt is then made to run one of the lymph strips a couple of centimetres into the irradiation area.

Because however some skin irritation occurs after a few days, there is a wait of two weeks before further extending the tape treatment. After this the taping causes no more problems and the scar of the right breast can also be taped.

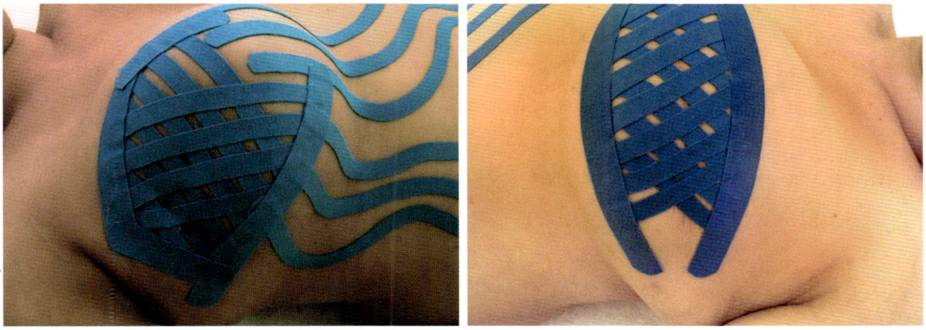

Photo left: right breast, crossed scar tape with three lymph strips from heterolateral inguinal and three lymph strips from homolateral inguinal ending on the caudal side and the medial side of the breast; further supplemented with four lymph strips from heterolateral axillary along the dorsal side to the lateral side of the breast – the latter is not shown in the photo.
Photo right: left breast, crossed scar tape The narrow ends of the scar tapes are additionally reinforced with a 2½ cm wide extra strip.
Width of the lymph strips: here ± 1.25 cm (5 cm wide tape cut into 4 strips); width of the strips of the scar tape: here ± 1 cm (5 cm wide tape cut into 5 strips)

Although the situation has clearly improved, there still remains a varying amount of lymph congestion present in the right breast, sometimes also with a slight increase in size of the right upper arm. The increase of lymphatic pressure seems to be clearly related to an increase in activity, and recovers when the activity is somewhat reduced.

Because of the varying situation the treatment is still continued, with a frequency of one treatment every seven to ten days.

This involves a genetically determined hormone-induced tumour where it is known that there is a high chance that the tumour will return in the breast not affected and the ovaries. For this reason initially the other breast is removed as a precaution and the ovaries will also be removed. The latter procedure follows three months after ending the radiotherapy.

After the ovaries have been removed via laparoscopy, there is again a post-operative increase in lymphatic pressure in the breast. At the same time there are some post-operative abdominal complaints. The treatment is adjusted for the situation.
Because of the abdominal complaints an anastomosis with tape from inguinal to the breast is not possible. If the lymphatic pressure from the breast is shifted to the abdomen, that could cause an increase in abdominal complaints.

Both on the left and right side four lymph strips are applied from the homolateral sternal region over the abdomen to prevent post-operative abdominal complaints.

The right breast is first taped with narrow tape strips from cranial to caudal, then longer lymph strips are applied from heterolateral axillary along the dorsal side to the right breast, where in the right breast a crossed lymph tape is applied.

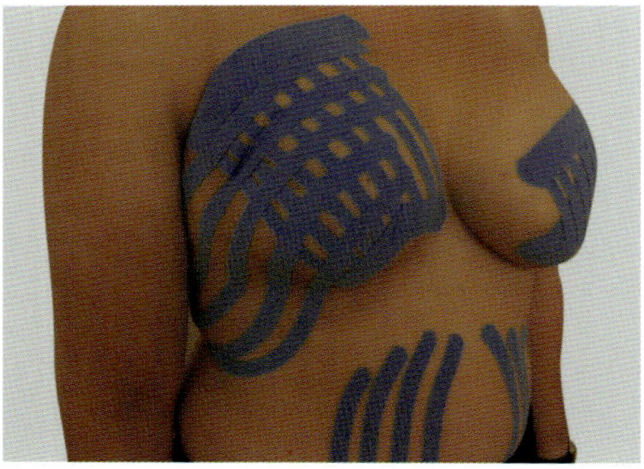

Bilateral parallel lymph strips from the sternal region over the abdomen; parallel local lymph strips over the right breast which are crossed by lymph strips from heterolateral axillary to the right breast.

Width of the lymph strips: here ± 1.25 cm (5 cm wide tape cut into 4 strips); the narrower local lymph strips on the right breast: here ± 0.8 cm (5 cm wide tape cut into 6 strips.

When the scars of the laparoscopy have healed and the abdominal complaints have disappeared again, the anastomosis tape from inguinal can be used again.

The treatment is continued as long as the lymph congestion in the right breast is still present. At the follow-up treatments an attempt is made to gradually reduce the treatment frequency and lower the intensity of the tape treatment. The tissue of both scars has become flexible and requires no further special attention.

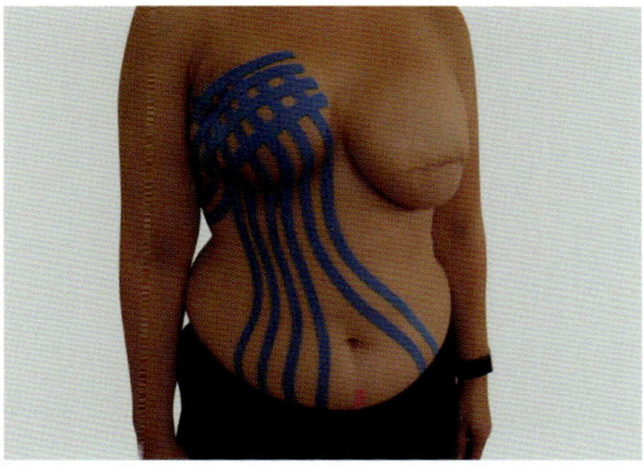

Seven months after starting the treatment: two lymph strips from heterolateral inguinal to the medial side of the breast, four lymph strips from homolateral inguinal to the middle and the lateral side of the breast, four lymph strips from heterolateral axillary via dorsal to the right breast. The lymph strips cross in the oedema area, where the treatment emphasis must lie.

Width of the lymph strips: here ± 1.25 cm (5 cm wide tape cut into 4 strips).

During the completion of this book this client is still under treatment.

6.3.3 Axillary node dissection, case 34

Case description:

A 43 year old housewife comes into the practice ten days after a mastectomy left, where a full axillary node dissection was also carried out. The operation was preceded by chemotherapy, radiotherapy will be started in around three weeks. She was referred to the practice because of a movement restriction in the left shoulder.

Upon examination a movement restriction glenohumeral in anteflexion and abduction direction is found. The maximum range of movement that can actively be achieved is restricted by the pain that occurs at the end of the movement in the armpit, where the scar has not yet healed.

There is a long scar, swelling is present particularly around the end points of the scar. There is no further palpable or visible oedema around the scar, the size of the left arm is slightly smaller compared with the right arm.

The first treatment consists only of manual lymph drainage. Five days later the second treatment follows. The range of movement glenohumeral is then already increased in anteflexion and abduction direction.

The second treatment also consists only of manual lymph drainage. Because of cognitive problems initially there is no treatment with a home exercise schedule, in the expectation that the range of movement will increase further when the scar has healed.

The therapy compliance of the client is poor, treatments are regularly cancelled. She comes back once more before the radiotherapy starts. There is then still a very slight movement restriction present, and still some swelling around the ends of the scar.

A week after the radiotherapy has started, she reports again to the practice. The irradiation effects are then already clearly visible and there is a developing lymphoedema in the irradiation area. Manual lymph drainage is carried out around the irradiation area. This treatment is supplemented with lymph tape, also around the irradiation area.

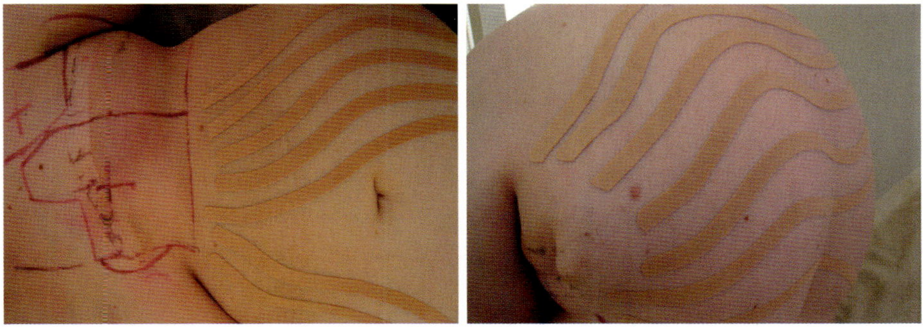

Situation one week after commencement of the radiotherapy. Lymph tape strips from homolateral and heterolateral inguinal to the caudal-ventral side of the irradiation area; from heterolateral axillary to the dorsolateral side of the irradiation area. Width of the lymph tape: here ± 1.25 cm (5 cm wide tape cut into 4 strips).

After this treatment the client cancels all treatments, she only comes for therapy again when the radiotherapy has ended. The lymphoedema in the irradiation area has then substantially increased and skin damage has occurred. The treatment with manual lymph drainage and lymph taping is then started again at a frequency of one treatment per week.

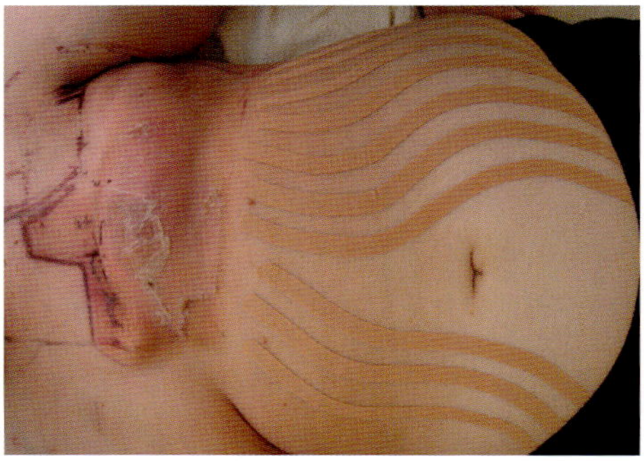

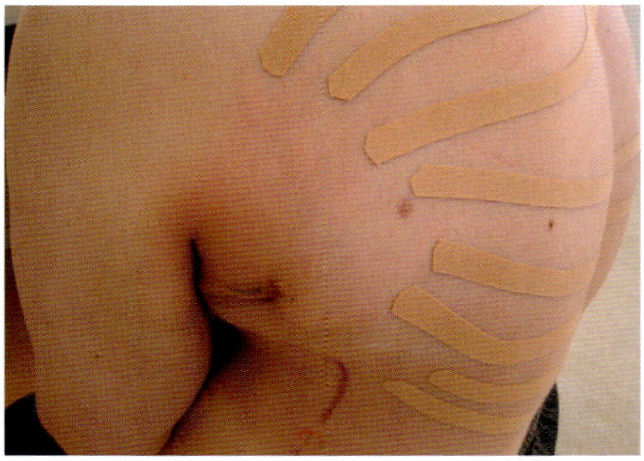

Situation just after ending the radiotherapy.
The lymph tape shown is similar to the above description.

After the radiotherapy has ended, the client does appear at every treatment appointment. The oedema is gradually reduced, after four weeks the dorsal tape strips are no longer applied because oedema is still only present on the ventral side.

The skin does however recover very slowly and seems not to be able to withstand any strain for a long time. Only after 10 weeks does the skin on the medial side of the scar appear to be sufficiently healed to allow the lymph tape strips to run a little further into the irradiation area. The lymph tape caudal from the scar on the ventral side is however repeated for each treatment.

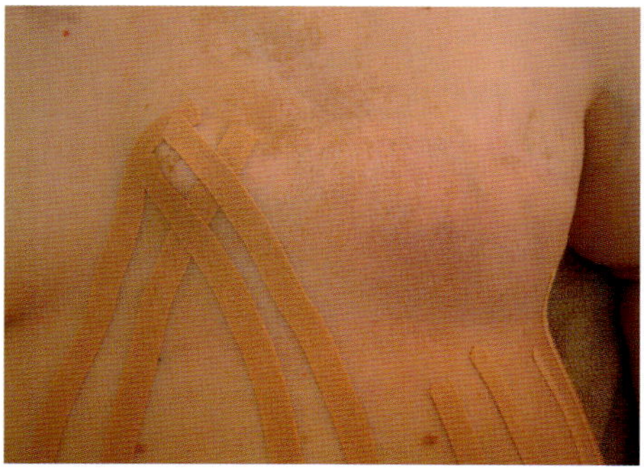

Ten weeks after ending the radiotherapy. The construction of the lymph tape is as described in the above photos, only on the medial side do the strips run a little further and cross over one another level with the medial end of the scar.

Upon the completion of this book this client is still in treatment.

6.4 Cervical lymph node dissection

After a cervical lymph node dissection the lymph drainage via the neck area is obstructed, which means that lymph congestion may occur in the face. Immediately after the operation the scar forms an additional obstruction to lymph drainage, the surface lymph vessels have been cut through and not yet regenerated. The effects of the irradiation can further obstruct lymph drainage from the face.

Once the scar is closed with skin, the tape treatment can be started, taking into account the restrictions that the radiotherapy can cause. (See also §5.7.4 and §6.2)

Because the physiological drainage path is obstructed to supraclavicular, the obvious choice is lymph taping with anastomoses. There are several possibilities for this.

Homolateral anastomoses are shown from paravertebral, from the axillary region and from parasternal. It is also possible to form an anastomosis from the inguinal region.

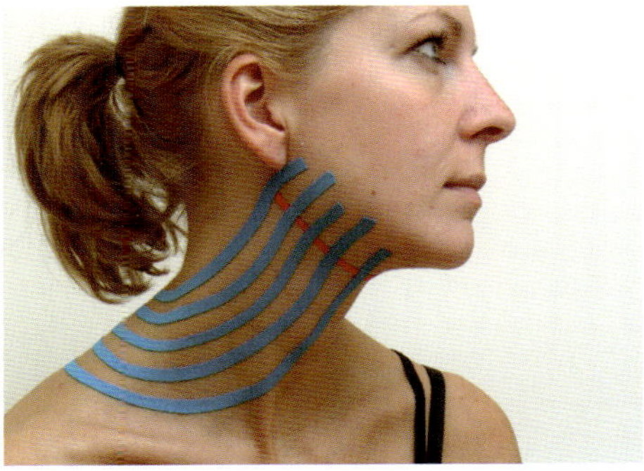

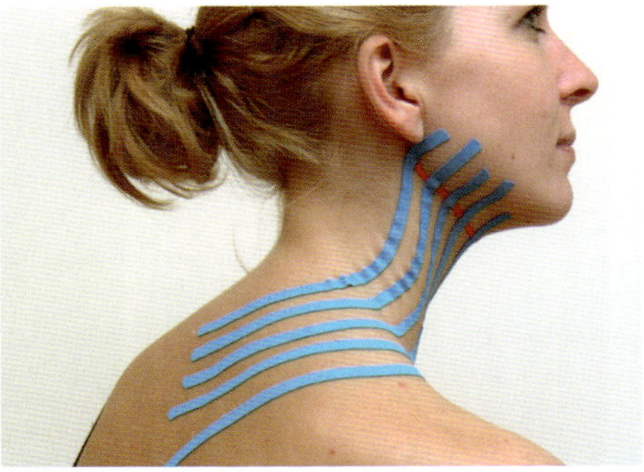

Parallel lymph strips from homolateral paravertebral to just over the scar, proximal from the problem area.
Width of the lymph strips: here ± 0.8 cm (5 cm wide tape cut into 6 strips).

If the problem is on both sides, the same tape method with homolateral anastomoses can be used for the other side of the face.

If the problem is on one side, then the lymph tape can be constructed from the heterolateral drainage areas, which gives more options.

In the figure the lymph tape is applied to just over the scar. When the lymphatic pressure in this area is reduced, the lymph can be drained more easily from the face.

If necessary or desirable, the lymph strips can also be applied a bit further into the face.

The treatment with parallel lymph strips can be made more intensive, by constructing extra anastomoses from another drainage area, which cross the first lymph strips.

For these crossing lymph strips the axillary region and the parasternal region are used here.

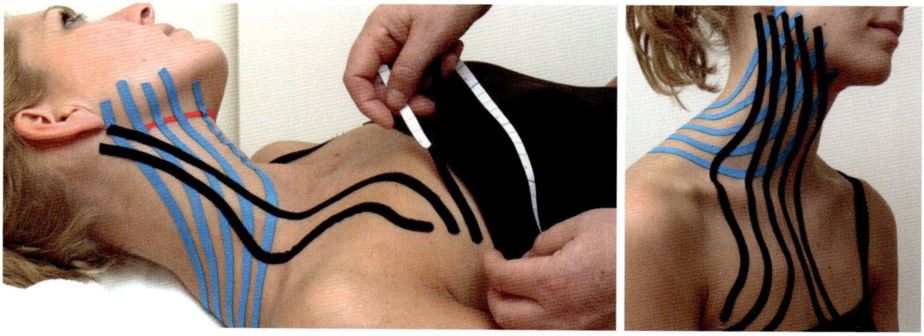

Crossing parallel lymph strips from homolateral axillary and homolateral parasternal to just over the scar, proximal from the problem area.
Width of the lymph strips: here ± 0.8 cm (5 cm wide tape cut into 6 strips).

By taping several anastomoses at the same time, an attempt is made to make the best possible use of the dispersion of the lymph congestion. The lymph will the most readily be drained to the area with the least flow resistance.

In the manual treatment the choice will often be anastomosis via the skull to the occipital edge. Due to the presence of head hair this anastomosis cannot be carried out with lymph tape.

In practice it regularly happens that certain theoretically possible anastomoses cannot be used.

If for example a client was involved here who in addition to the problem described also suffers from orthopaedic symptoms low cervical or high thoracic, then the lymph tape from paravertebral could cause increased pressure in the vertebrae which could further increase the orthopaedic symptoms. In that case another anastomosis must be chosen.

N.B. The possible scar is indicated in the photos with a narrow strip of pink tape.

6.4.1 Correlation secondary lymphoedema? Case 33

Case description:

A 61 year old female teacher comes into the practice because of pain symptoms in the lower arm and hand after a fracture in the processus styloideus of the radius left. The fracture occurred three weeks before, but was not identified as such at the GP surgery. It was only a week later that an X-ray was taken, after which the wrist was immobilised with a plaster.
In the past two weeks increasing pain symptoms have occurred in the lower arm and in the hand. Because of the pain symptoms the plaster has already been checked and replaced twice, but this has had no effect on the pain.

When she comes into the practice, she has continuous pain. The symptoms increase at night, there is then a tight and heavy feeling in the lower arm, which she describes as the pressure of a sphygmanometer.
The size of the left upper arm has not visibly, measurably or palpably increased compared with the right upper arm. The fingers of the left hand are however rather swollen compared with the fingers of the right hand. Stemmer's test is positive for the fingers of the left hand, but not on the right side.

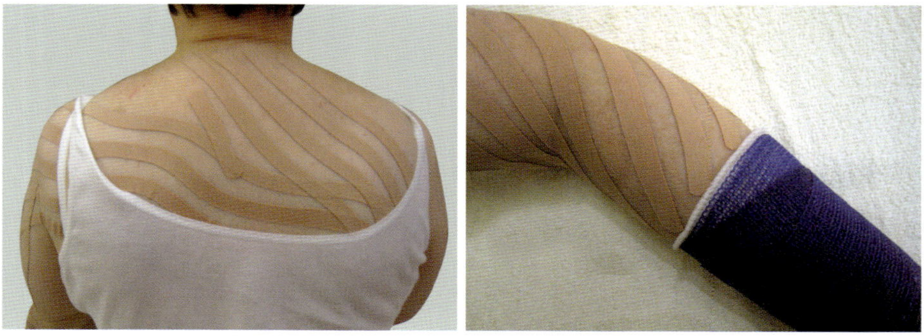

Parallel lymph strips from heterolateral axillary via dorsal to the left arm, ending on the upper edge of the plaster; combined with parallel lymph strips from axillary right to the CTJ.

Width of the lymph strips: here ± 1.25 cm (5 cm wide tape cut into 4 strips).

From the history it is known that ten years ago she had skin cancer in the face. The cancer was surgically removed and then treated with radiotherapy on the left side of the face and neck. During the radiotherapy period an erysipelas infection occurred five times in the irradiation area. No lymph nodes were removed during the operation.Furthermore she has regular neck symptoms, which emerges when in the inspection a thickening around the cervico thoracic transition is noticed. At the time of the treatment she has no neck symptoms.

Because of the increased lymphatic pressure the treatment is started with lymph tape. Because of the history and the latent neck symptoms present, an anastomosis is used here. From heterolateral axillary parallel lymph strips are applied to the left arm. The lymph strips end just by the upper edge of the plaster. Also to relieve the CTJ area, subsequently a few more lymph strips are applied from axillary right to the CTJ area. By applying the lymph tape in this way, an attempt is made as far as possible to avoid the left supraclavicular region.

Because a developing dystrophy cannot be excluded, after 24 hours there is a telephone consultation. At that time the pain symptoms already appear to have reduced somewhat and the heavy feeling at night was much less clearly present.

Two days later she says that she is tolerating the tape very badly and has meanwhile removed most of it. The heavy feeling in the lower arm has gone, but has now moved to the upper arm. It makes her rather uncertain and she in fact first wants to seek the advice of the treating specialist. After this she decided on another treatment process and has not been back to the practice again. *

Because of the history this case is included in the chapter secondary oedema, although in fact there seems not to be any secondary oedema. It is possible that the symptom pattern after the fracture is completely unrelated to the cancer and the subsequent treatment of ten years ago. It is however also possible that the drainage capacity of the lymphatic system was reduced by the radiotherapy and the erysipelas on the left side.

The lymph tape treatment is therefore constructed as if the drainage capacity on the left side was in fact actually reduced. This is also the reason for still including this case in this chapter.

**On contact six weeks later it appears the size of hand and fingers has increased and a dystrophy has developed.*

6.5 Groin lymph node dissection

After a resection of the inguinal lymph nodes oedema may occur in all areas that would normally drain the lymph via these lymph nodes. In the case of a unilateral resection there is chance of lymph congestion in the homolateral leg, the homolateral-caudal quadrant of the abdomen and the homolateral genital area.

Because the lymphatic system by its very nature has alternative drainage possibilities, the problem of lymph congestion does not have to arise. But the chance of lymphoedema occurring continues to exist for the rest of the life, even if there have been no symptoms for years after the procedure. Immediately after the operation the scar can form an additional obstacle to lymph drainage, the surface lymph vessels have been cut through and not yet regenerated. The effects of any radiotherapy may further hinder lymph drainage.

Once the scar is closed with skin, tape treatment can be started over the scar, taking into account the restrictions that radiotherapy may cause (see also §5.7.4 and §6.2). Before the scar is completely closed, it is however possible to tape round the scar.

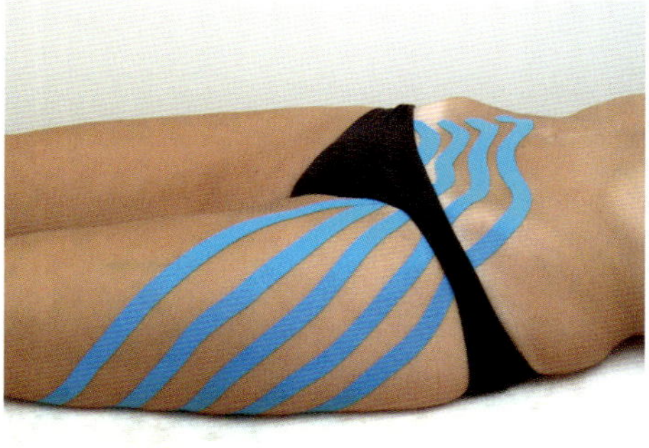

Parallel lymph strips from the heterolateral groin/lower abdomen, via ventral to the upper leg.
Width of the lymph strips: here ± 1.25 cm (5 cm wide tape cut into 4 strips).

Because there is a functional restriction of the natural drainage path, the obvious choice during the treatment is a tape construction with anastomoses.

In the case of a unilateral problem the anastomoses can be constructed from the heterolateral lower abdomen or groin area, from sternal, from paravertebral, from homolateral axillary or even from heterolateral axillary.

Here an example is shown of a unilateral problem. The lymph strips can run without interruption into the area with oedema, or, depending on the treatment construction, as far as is required.

In the example only the upper leg is treated with tape. If the lower leg and foot also have to be taped, the strips can be applied up to the dorsum of the foot. The exception made for the hand, does not apply for the foot.

If more lymph strips are necessary, then these can possibly be 'attached' to a previous strip. A spread of these attachment points is required. If too many bases of lymph strips are applied to one and the same point, the tape will work loose sooner at that concentration point. Furthermore the tape construction is then comparable with a lymph tape in the fan-shaped model.

The treatment can be intensified by using more lymph strips and/or by working with several anastomoses at the same time.

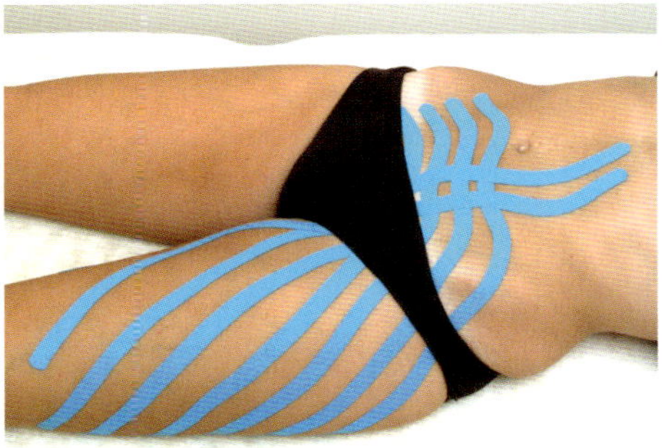

Parallel lymph strips from the heterolateral groin/lower abdomen, via ventral to the upper leg, supplemented with parallel lymph strips from sternal.
Width of the lymph strips: here ± 1.25 cm (5 cm wide tape cut into 4 strips).

By applying a lymph tape with crossing lymph strips from other anastomosis sites, the treatment is even more intensive. Such intensive treatment is not always necessary and is also not always well tolerated, but can in certain cases be a good treatment method.

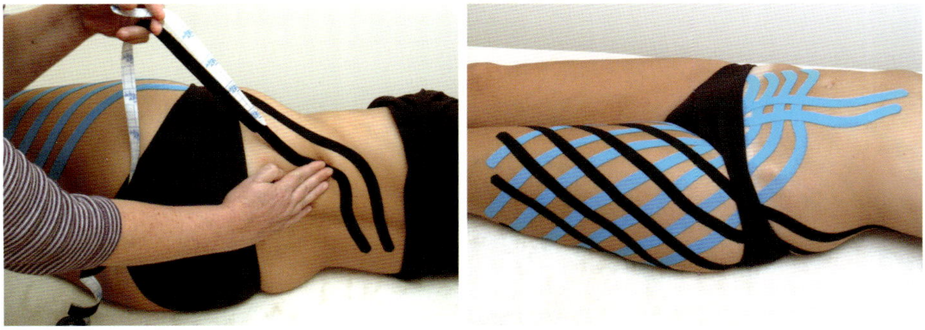

Parallel lymph strips from the heterolateral groin/lower abdomen and parallel lymph strips from sternal, crossed by parallel lymph strips from heterolateral paravertebral.
Width of the lymph strips: here ± 1.25 cm (5 cm wide tape cut into 4 strips).

In the case of bilateral resection of the lymph nodes there is of course a chance of lymph congestion on both the left and right side. The anastomosis to the heterolateral lower abdomen or to the heterolateral inguinal region cannot then be used.

In that case the choice may be for an anastomosis from sternal, an anastomosis from paravertebral or an anastomosis from axillary. A combination of these anastomoses is also possible. It seems logical in case of such a problem to tape from the homolateral side (see also the description in § 7.2).

6.5.1 Genital oedema

A genital oedema can be treated with tape by positioning the lymph strips from a drainage area to the genital area, where the strips end as close as possible to the oedema. By stimulating lymph drainage as far as possible proximal from the oedema, the lymphatic pressure in the proximal area will be reduced. The lymph accumulation in the oedema will as a result move more easily to the area with the lower pressure and in this way can be further reduced.

Various drainage paths are possible for genital oedema. An anastomosis can be made from sternal, from paravertebral or from axillary. A combination is also possible.

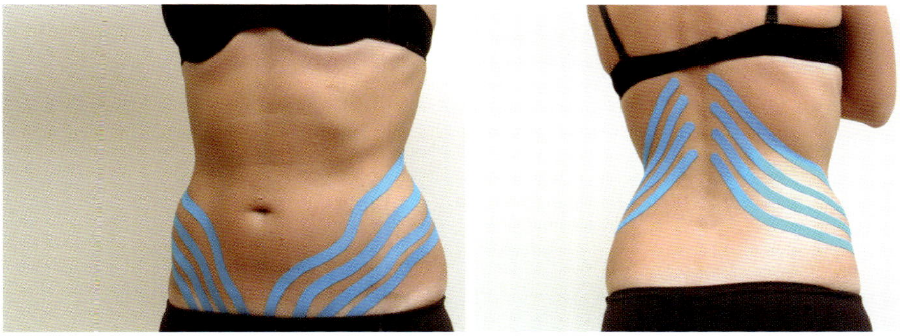

Bilateral, parallel lymph strips from homolateral paravertebral, ending level with the os pubis, just proximal from the genital oedema.
Width of the lymph strips: here ± 1.25 cm (5 cm wide tape cut into 4 strips).

It may happen that both legs must be treated with lymph tape and a genital oedema at the same time. The possible anastomoses can then be spread out, so that a combination arises. For example parallel lymph strips from sternal to the os pubis for the genital oedema, combined with parallel lymph strips from homolateral paravertebral that are applied into the homolateral leg.

6.6 Diaphragm / gastric area

This extra paragraph is included because the segmental tape presented here can considerably reduce or even completely eliminate the nausea that may occur during chemotherapy.

Required tape	two strips of tape, 5 cm wide.
Measure tape 1	measure in stretched position, caudal from the processus xiphoideus, over almost the whole width of the trunk.
Measure tape 2	measure in stretched position level with Th12, over almost the whole width of the trunk.
Technique	standard technique, stretch on the skin, no extra stretch on the tape.
Apply tape 1	the skin is stretched by anteflexion of the arms and breathing in to maximum, after which the tape is positioned caudal from the processus xiphoideus to lateral. The anchors are applied in the neutral position.
Apply tape 2	the skin is stretched by protraction of the shoulder girdle, flexion in the spine and maximum inhalation. After this the tape is applied at the level of Th12 to lateral. The anchors are applied in the neutral position.
Tape direction	from the middle to lateral.

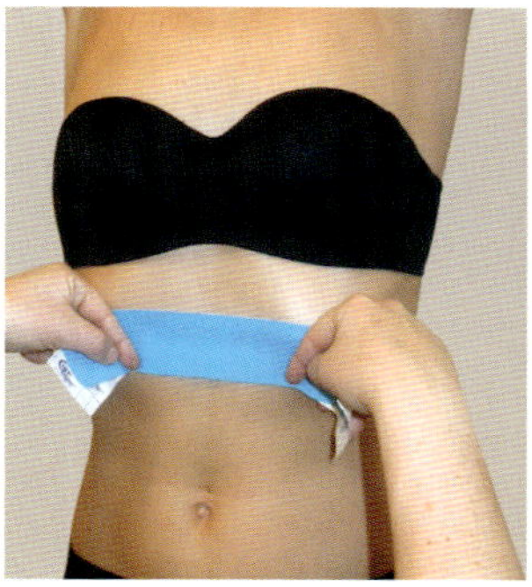

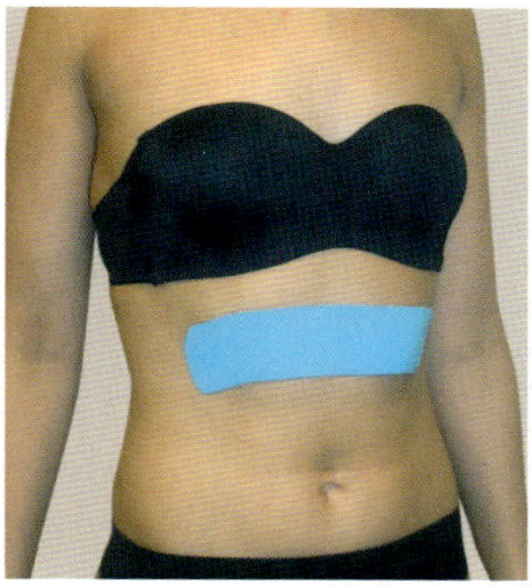

Tape 1.

This tape is applied in the dermatome Th7/Th8.

The diaphragm is innervated from C2 to C4 inclusive. The parasympathetic innervation of the stomach is supplied from C2 to C4 inclusive, the sympathetic innervation is supplied from Th5 to Th9 inclusive.

Both from the dermatome and from the innervation of the diaphragm there is then a segmental relation with the stomach.

A small part of the tape is located in the ventral gastric area as described by Piët, Sachs and Sachs-Piët. The ventral gastric zone is located on the left side of the body in a triangle bordered by the median line and the costal margin, just caudal from the processus xiphoideus.

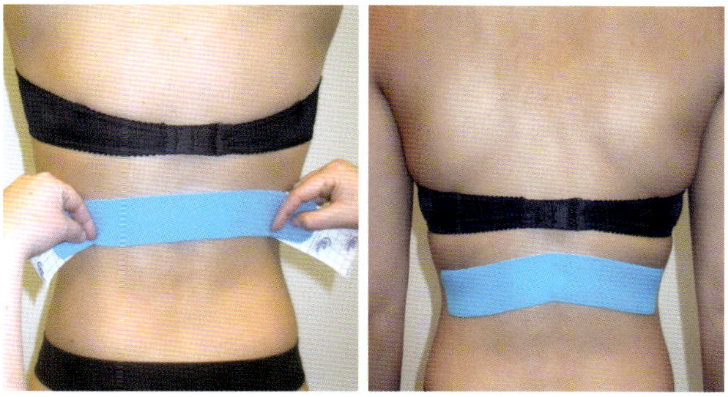

Tape 2.

This tape is applied in the dermatome Th8/Th9. The diaphragm is innervated from C2 to C4 inclusive. The parasympathetic innervation of the stomach is supplied from C2 to C4 inclusive, the sympathetic innervation is supplied from Th5 to Th9 inclusive.

Both from the dermatome and from the innervation of the diaphragm there is then a segmental relation with the stomach.
A minimal part of the tape is located in the dorsal gastric area as described by Piët, Sachs and Sachs-Piët. The dorsal gastric zone is located on the left side of the body, bordered at the top by the shoulder blade and on the underside bordered by the costal margin.

7. Primary lymphoedema and lipo-lymphoedema

7.1 Introduction

Although primary lymphoedema, lipoedema and lipo-lymphoedema are differently defined (see §3.4.1 and §3.5.1), these disorders are still summarised within this chapter. Because in the case of lipoedema deviations in the lymph vessels are also described that cause reduced functionality, this combination seems a natural one.

Furthermore, primary lymphoedema and lipoedema in certain cases seem to be difficult to distinguish (see §7.2, case 3). Furthermore the distinction between lipoedema and primary lymphoedema has no consequences for treatment with lymph taping, but it does for the rules for life and dietary rules.

Comments on the advantages and disadvantages of lymph taping are similar to the comments made in §6.1. If compression therapy can be replaced by treatment with lymph taping, this means a considerable improvement in the quality of life.

For small children, such as the little girl whose case is described in §7.3, lymph taping can offer a very important solution. The child can move around as normal with the lymph tapes and is even hampered less by this because the oedema is reduced. That this is essential for the development of the child needs no further argument.

7.2 Primary lymphoedema, case 3

Case description:

At the age of 16 years this woman was diagnosed with bilateral primary lymphoedema based on a lymph scintigraphy, with distichiasis as an additional characteristic. Over 6 years later the condition was named as lipoedema by another specialist. After this she had two surgical procedures in which lympho-venous shunts were made. This had no result, after which lymphosuction was carried out. The latter procedure also gave no improvement.

Since then she has permanently painful legs. She has already been treated for years with manual lymph drainage at a frequency of at least once a week. She wears elastic stockings class 3 to the groin, without these stockings the symptoms increase considerably. Because the treatment with the oedema therapist is very painful, she has had no further treatment in recent months before she came into the practice.

Four years after the last operation she reports to the practice because she has heard of the possibilities of treatment with lymph taping. She would like to try out whether in this way she would have to wear her compression stockings less frequently.

At the first treatment she is suffering mainly from a heavy, painful feeling on the medial and the ventral side of both knees. Stemmer's test is positive in both feet and to a lesser extent positive in the fingers of both hands. There is moderate oedema present in upper legs and lower legs that feels soft, but is already non-pitting.

The treatment starts with manual lymph drainage, followed by tape treatment. Because the abdominal region still feels sensitive during manual treatment, the lymph tapes are positioned from paravertebral.

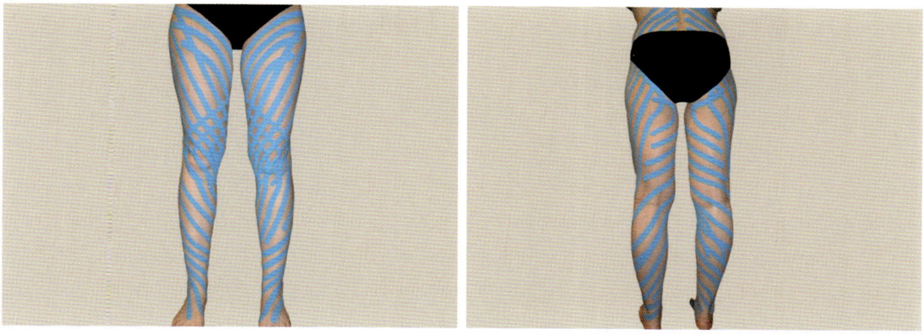

Parallel local lymph strips from cranio-medial upper leg to the ventral and medial side of the patella; the local strips are crossed by parallel lymph strips from homolateral paravertebral which run spirally as far as the foot.
Width of the tape strips: the local short strips ± 1 cm wide (5 cm wide tape cut into 4 strips), the long strips ± 1.25 cm wide (5 cm wide tape cut into 4 strips).

At the start of the second treatment she is enthusiastic, she has not had to wear compression stockings the whole week. The evening prior to the second treatment she removed the tape and on the treatment day she did not wear her compression stockings, so that at the time of the treatment there is an increase in symptoms. The second treatment is carried out in accordance with the first treatment.

The treatments continue well for a time, but after a number of months tape irritation suddenly seems to occur. The reason for this tape irritation is not entirely clear. The summer outside temperatures could have something to do with this, but it is also clear that the original tape product has changed in quality.

In any case it is not possible to tape over the irritated skin and she is forced to wear compression stockings until the skin has recovered. Because the skin irritation is mainly present around the knees, taping is possible on the proximal side of the stocking. At the same time another tape product is used (CureTape), which seems to be of a better quality.

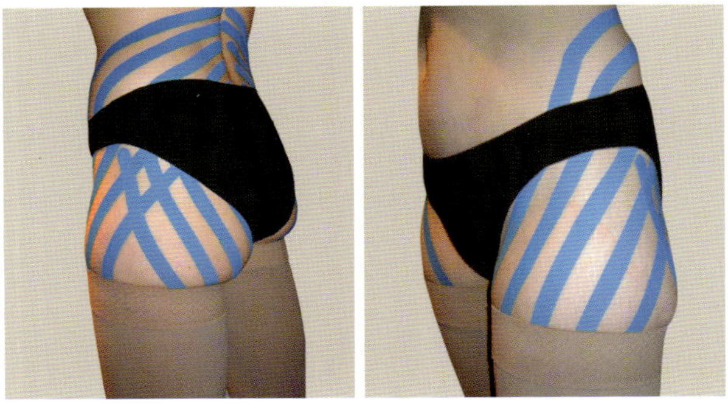

Parallel lymph strips from paravertebral ending just under the upper edge of the compression stockings.
Width of the tape strips: here ± 1.25 cm wide (5 cm wide tape cut into 4 strips).

The new product does in fact appear to be of a better quality. After two weeks the tape irritation has disappeared and the lymph tape treatment can be continued again.

In the following months she is treated weekly. The treatments go reasonably similar to the first treatment, although from time to time other methods of applying the tape are tried out. In one of these treatments a very solid tape is applied, with long parallel strips from high paravertebral in a spiral to the foot, crossing with long parallel strips from sternal. This lymph tape is supplemented with orthopaedic tapes around the knee.

During the evaluation at the start of the next treatment, it is found that this approach was probably too intensive. After three days she has removed the tape because of an increase in symptoms. The rest of the week she has worn her compression stockings again.
In consultation it is decided to use markedly less intensive taping and only to use parallel lymph strips from sternal to the knee, in combination with compression stockings to the knee.

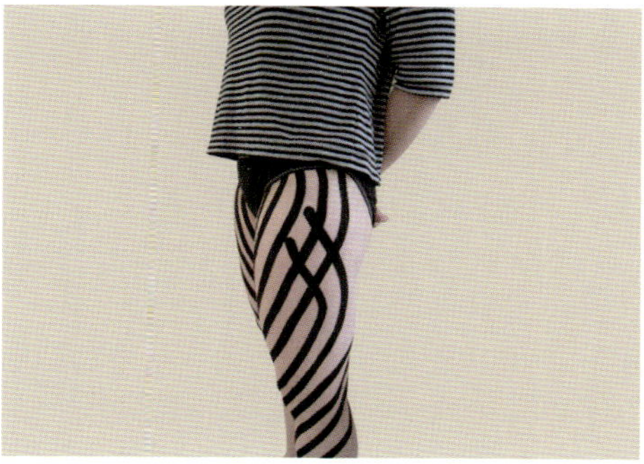
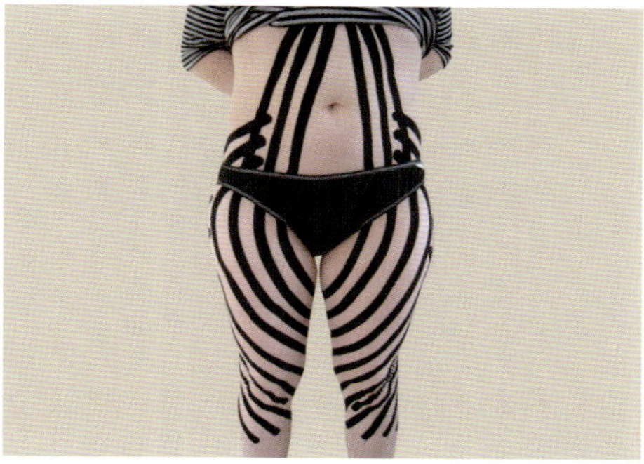

Parallel lymph strips from sternal to just peripheral from the knees, subsequently combined with compression stockings to the knee.
Width of the tape strips: here ± 1.25 cm wide (5 cm wide tape cut into 4 strips).

The method appears to be successful and the treatment is continued in this way. It soon appears that the compression stockings to the knee do not in fact add very much, after which she leaves off the compression stockings. Because the method is very satisfactory, no changes are tried for a long time after this.

In a period in which lumbar symptoms are combined with some abdominal complaints, the tape method is adapted to the current situation. The lymph tape strips are then applied from high thoracic paravertebral to the abdomen, and from the abdomen in a spiral to the knees.

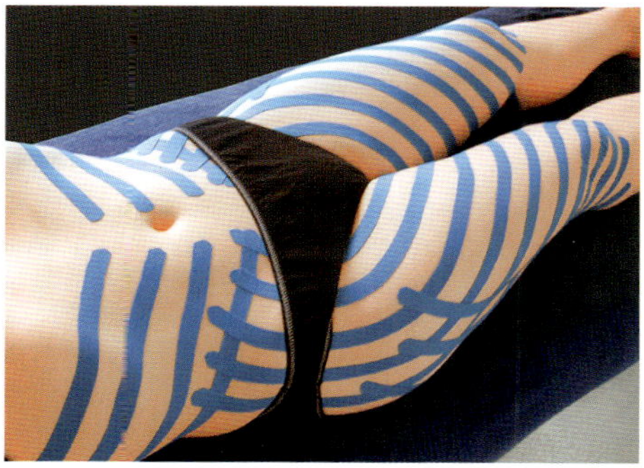

Parallel lymph tape strips from high thoracic paravertebral to the abdomen, from the abdomen in a spiral to the knees.
Width of the tape strips: here ± 1.25 cm wide (5 cm wide tape cut into 4 strips).

In the photos the spiral tapes always run to medial. The lymph tape strips were also applied in a spiral to lateral, but this gave a subjectively less good treatment result. Within our own practice this client is the only one who has a pronounced preference for lymph strips that run to medial.

In the course of time more vertically running lymph tapes and lymph tapes applied in a wave have been tried, but both gave a subjectively less good treatment result. However the angle of inclination of the lymph tape strips has changed somewhat and at present the tape is applied in more gradual spirals.

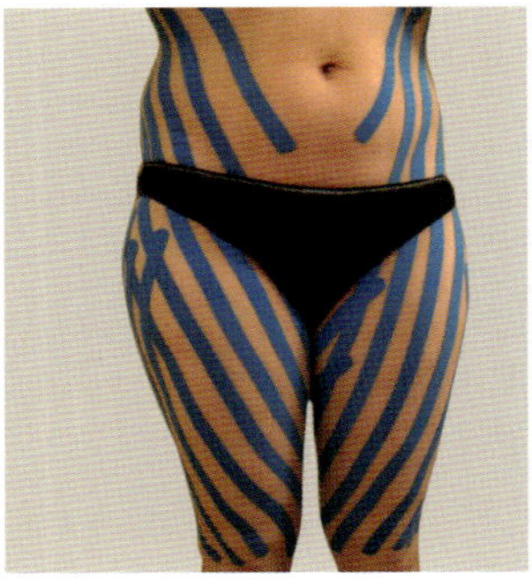

Parallel lymph strips from axillary in gradual spirals to the knee.
Width of the tape strips: here ± 1.25 cm wide (5 cm wide tape cut into 4 strips).

With these lymph tapes the client has remained stable over the last five years on average. Occasionally there is a temporary increase in volume and symptoms, usually attributable to known causes. She is in principle treated weekly with manual lymph drainage and lymph tape. If a treatment is cancelled, the client tapes herself at home. She no longer uses compression stockings.

7.3 Turner syndrome, case 22

Case description:

This, now 14 month old, little girl has Turner syndrome. Immediately after birth there was already clear lymphoedema visible in the arms and legs.

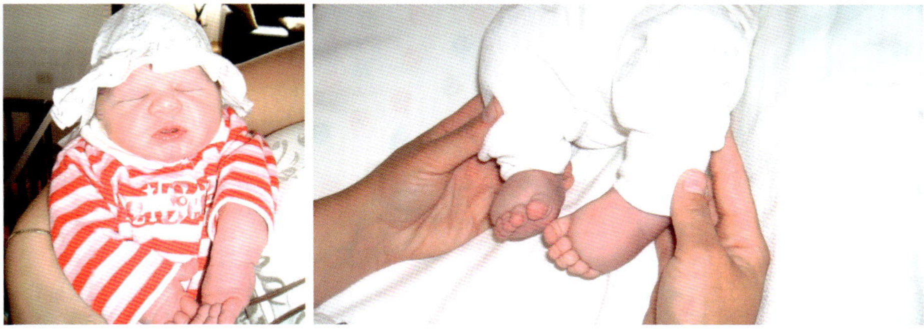

Lymphoedema post partum.

During the first year of life the little girl was seen by many therapists, including an oedema therapist. The treatments with manual lymph drainage have a good result. Because of the improved situation and because of the treatment pressure, this treatment is discontinued in the course of time.

In the following period the lymphoedema builds up again. The mother would like to try and see whether this can be treated using lymph taping. The little girl has a lot of experience with therapists and is plainly inconsolable as soon as she understands that she is being taken near therapists. The intention is then also to try one treatment and if the result is positive to then instruct the mother, so that she can tape the little girl herself at home.

The lymphoedema is mainly visibly present in the arms and the legs. Furthermore the little girl has a lot of itching on her body and she starts to scratch as soon as her clothes are taken off. Because both arms and both legs show lymphoedema, it is decided to apply lymph tape to all the extremities from homolateral paravertebral.

In order to upset the little girl as little as possible, an attempt is made to keep the treatment intensity as low as possible. Narrow strips are used that are not made too long, but end in the proximal part of the extremities.

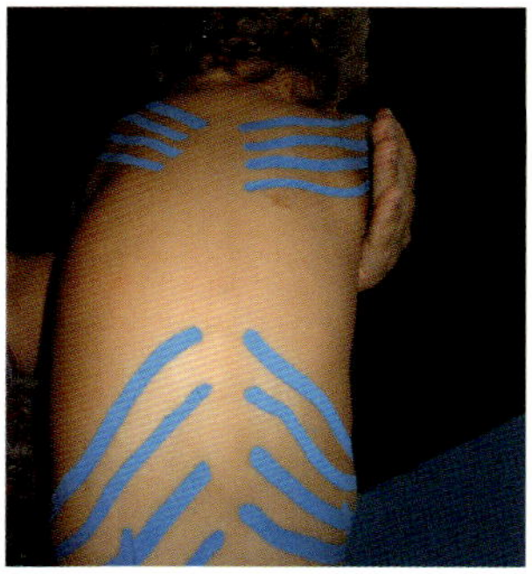

Parallel lymph tape from homolateral thoracic ending in the upper arms; from homolateral lower thoracic/ lumbar ending in the upper legs.
Width of the tape strips: here ± 0.8 cm (5 cm wide tape cut into 6 strips).

At the second meeting this approach appears to be successful, also peripherally there is a clear volume reduction. In addition the itching appeared to have clearly reduced during the time that she was taped.

The mother has been taught to apply the tape correctly and she now treats the little girl with CureTape herself as soon as the situation requires this. During the last follow-up this home treatment appears to be going extremely well.

7.4 Lipo-lymphoedema, case 36

Case description:

This 32 year old manager is diagnosed with lipoedema and with hypermobility syndrome, as a result of which she has varying symptoms in her joints. In particular the knees give symptoms, but in case of stress the other joints can also give many symptoms. She has reported to the practice because of these joint symptoms. The symptoms already appear to have existed for years and to have begun around adolescence. The diagnosis of HMS was made about seven years ago, the diagnosis of lipoedema is very recent.

As an adolescent and young adult she played top level korfball. When this could no longer be combined with her professional work, she started intensive fitness training. In spite of practising sport intensively which was regularly accompanied by strict dieting, the size of her legs increased. Until the diagnosis of lipoedema was made, these symptoms were not understood and/or not pointed out (see § 3.4.1 and § 3.5.1).

The volume in the left leg is somewhat greater than the volume in the right leg. Stemmer's sign is positive in both feet. From this the conclusion was drawn that lipo-lymphoedema is present. The explanation of this condition explains to her a lot about the previous process.

Manual lymph drainage is started. In combination with clear rules for life and moderate exercise the situation seems to stabilise and she is also symptom free for lengthy periods.

.

Due to increasing pressure at work she is forced to discontinue the treatment in the practice for a while. When she comes back into the practice after four months, she has a lot of pain symptoms in her knees and to a lesser extent in her wrists. The treatment with manual lymph drainage is resumed and supported with lymph tape treatment.

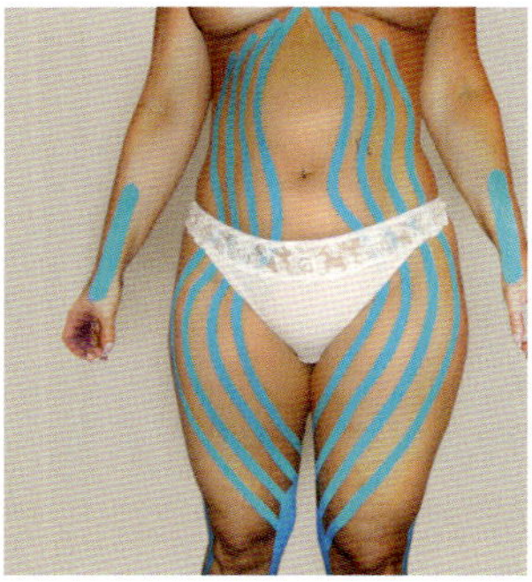

Parallel lymph strips from central to the medial side of the knees, combined with orthopaedic stabilising tapes on the knees and wrists.
Width of the lymph tape: here ± 1.25 cm wide (5 cm wide tape cut into 4 strips).

After three treatments the joint symptoms have reduced again. The lymph tape treatment is reduced and the treatment continues further according to the previously drawn up treatment plan with manual lymph drainage at a low frequency, rules for life and moderate exercise therapy.

Bibliography

Bernards J.A. & Bouman L.N., Fysiologie van de mens, Utrecht, Bohn Scheltema & Holkema, 1979

Bringezu G. & Schreiner O., Lehrbuch der Entstauungstherapie, Heidelberg, Springer, 2006

Cranenburgh B. van, Segmentale Verschijnselen, Houten, Bohn Stafleu van Loghum, 1998

Damstra Drs. R.J. et al, Richtlijn Lymfoedeem,Alphen aan den Rijn, van Zuiden, 2002

Damstra Dr. R.J., Diagnostic and Therapeutical Aspects of Lymphedema, Drachten, SLCN, 2009

Földi M., Földi E., Kubik S., Lehrbuch der Lymphologie, München, Elsevier, 2005

Kasseroller R., Kompendium der Manuellen Lymphdrainage nach Dr. Vodder, Heidelberg, Haug, 1996

Kenzo K. et al, Kinesio Taping for Lymphoedema and Chronic Swelling, Kinesio USA, 2006

Lohman A H.M., Vorm en Beweging, Utrecht, Bohn Scheltema & Holkema, 1980,

Platzer W. Atlas van de Anatomie, Baarn, Bosch & Keuning, 1981

Piët J.F.M , Sachs J.J., Sachs-Piët I.M.A., Bindweefselmassage, Maarsen, Elsevier/De Tijdstroom, 1999

Pijnappel H., Medical Taping Concept Handbook, Tapingbase, 2009

Sijmonsma J., Medical Taping Concept Manual, Goor, Fysionair, 2004

Sobotta J. en Becher H., Atlas der Anatomie des Menschen – vol.1, Berlijn, Urban&Schwartzenberg, 1972

Teirich-Leube H., Grondbeginselen van de bindweefselmassage, Lochem-Poperinge, De Tijdstroom, 1979

Verdonk H.P.M., Oedeem en oedeemtherapie, Houten, Bohn Stafleu van Loghum, 2000

Weissleder H. & Schuchhardt C., Erkrankungen des Lymphgefä systems, Essen, Viavital, 2006

Wittlinger H. & Wittlinger G., Lehrbuch der Manuellen Lymphdrainage nach Dr. vodder – vol.2, Heidelberg, Haug, 1996

Zuther J. E., Lymphedema Management, New York, Thieme, 2005

Index

D

E

F

G

H

M

N